Troubleshooting the Mind

Understanding the
Basic Principles of the Kelee®

TROUBLESHOOTING THE MIND
Understanding the Basic Principles of the Kelee®

This book is an original publication of Quiescence Publishing

PRINTING HISTORY
first edition / June 2010

www.thekelee.org

ISBN: 978-0-9973002-3-9

PRINTED IN THE UNITED STATES OF AMERICA

Acknowledgements

There are many people I would like to thank...

My mentor, Dr. Eugene C. Larr, who introduced me to the Kelee in 1985 and who I consulted with as new discoveries of the Kelee came to light.

Lavana Rathbun, CFO of the Kelee Foundation, for her support, patience, and love over the years as each day unfolded into the next.

Nikki Walsh, MBA, for all of her diligence and behind-the-scenes efforts in laying the groundwork of the Kelee Foundation, Quiescence Publishing, and the medical study.

Dr. Daniel Lee for starting the medical study at the University of California, San Diego Medical Center and for being open to seeing how profound and invaluable the knowledge of the Kelee is to medicine.

Dr. Amy Sitapati for her innate awareness of the Kelee, its importance, and her willingness to help bring the medical study about.

Frank Silva, MPH, for his input on this book and eagerness to teach the Practice.

Moira Mar-Tang, MPH, for the countless hours she has donated to help with the medical study.

There are many others who have freely offered their time and energy because they know it is important to the future of our planet to understand the difference between brain and mind.

To troubleshoot the mind,
you must have a way.
That way is found through
a practical understanding of
how to still the mind on command.
It is from a still mind
that all can be seen clearly.

—Ron W. Rathbun

Contents

Relax the mind, heal the body;
this truth is profoundly deep
when you can feel it for yourself.
Do you know how to relax your mind
and how often do you do it?

—Ron W. Rathbun

Foreword

By Daniel Lee, MD

You may be asking yourself, "Why should I try Kelee meditation (or the "Practice" as it is known amongst those who already do it)?" The answer to this question is both simple and complex. Before answering this question, ask yourself the following: Do you truly want to feel better both mentally and physically? If your answer is yes, then Kelee meditation is your road map in learning how you can feel better and how you can improve your own quality of life.

Kelee meditation is a way for you to learn about yourself—your own thoughts and your own feelings. What could be more interesting or more important to you than what you think or what you feel in your life every day? However, how much time do we spend paying attention to our thoughts or our feelings?

If you were like me, probably not much time at all. We tend to only look at our own thoughts and feelings when we are forced to—usually by painful events in our own lives.

Pain, whether mental or physical, often makes us stop and reevaluate our life. This was certainly the case for me. An unexpected breakup in my relationship had occurred, and I was forced to look at all of the negative thoughts and feelings I had inside of me. It was then that I started Kelee meditation to help me calm my endless brain chatter and to understand for myself why I was in pain.

Have you ever noticed how much brain chatter we all have throughout the day? If you pay attention to this mindless chatter, you will notice that these thoughts are usually either negative or unresolved, which is why they tend to stay on our mind. So what is the effect of negative thoughts?

As a physician, I have seen how negative thoughts affect many of my patients, as well as myself. Negative thoughts can cause tension in the physical body, which can manifest in many different ways, such as the development of stomach aches, headaches, and muscle tightness in the neck and/or back.

Over time, severe medical conditions, such as high blood pressure, heart disease, and cancer can develop. It is interesting that an emphasis of the medical profession is preventative health, yet we spend very little time proactively to understand our own thoughts and feelings, which can clearly affect our health and quality of life.

When we have all of this mindless brain chatter, we can

often feel distracted, unfocused, worried, and stressed. Kelee meditation, as you will learn, is focused on stillness of the mind, which will help with calming the chatter in the brain. This will lead directly to a feeling of peace and calmness, and over time translates to improved natural focus and being in mind.

When you have fewer negative and/or unresolved thoughts and worries, you become less anxious and stressed. You will also begin to notice improved clarity of perception and self-awareness. Kelee meditation will allow you to experience peace of mind, the feeling of contentment, and true freedom from what weighs you down.

While Kelee meditation starts as a meditation technique for you to learn how to quiet your own brain chatter, it really is a way for you to understand your own mind. Kelee meditation is not a belief system, nor is it associated with a particular type of religion. Kelee meditation will help you to understand why you have taken in and accepted negative thoughts and feelings, and provides a way for you to truly get rid of them forever.

Many of us often try to cope with life when things do not go our way. Some may turn to drugs and alcohol to escape from the pain, while others seek healthier solutions to cope with pain. However, Kelee meditation is especially unique in that it does not teach you how to cope with a situation, but instead how to eliminate the underlying trigger that is causing your pain. All that is required is 5 to 10 minutes twice a day of practicing stilling your mind.

So why should you try Kelee meditation? As I have

stated, there is a simple answer as well as a complex answer. I have just given you the short, simple, intellectual answer from my own personal experience. Kelee meditation has certainly transformed my life and the way I think and feel about my life. The following pages outline the intellectual understanding of the Kelee—from how to do the meditation practice to how stillness of mind leads to the positive effects of Kelee meditation.

However, life is really about direct experience—not just secondhand intellectual knowledge. The complex answer as to why you should try Kelee meditation is waiting for you to experience. Once you've experienced this for yourself, you will glimpse an understanding of the enormous unlimited potential of what Kelee meditation can do for you. So what do you have to lose by trying Kelee meditation? Just negativity and discontentment. Try Kelee meditation for yourself and truly experience life.

Daniel Lee, MD
Associate Clinical Professor of Medicine
UCSD School of Medicine
UCSD Medical Center—Owen Clinic
January 2010

*The feeling in your mind fuels
the feeling in your body.
When your mind
is growing and learning,
it is that feeling
that manifests health and healing.*

—Ron W. Rathbun

If you are not paying attention to your health, who is responsible for it? When you realize that your thoughts affect your mental and physical well-being, you will have another way to improve your health.

Introduction

Kelee meditation was founded over two decades of research by a process of observing what works. It is not a theory; it is an understanding of the mind and simply put, it is the way it is. The basic principles in this book are all you need to get started to heal yourself on psychological and physiological levels. There is nothing in the physical body that the mind does not control. What can you do without your mind?

Have you ever noticed that when you feel bad mentally, you never feel good physically? This is because the mind runs the central nervous system, which runs the physical body. Everyone at one time or another has had a negative thought that upset his or her stomach. This is an example of when psychology has affected the physiology of the body. If negative thoughts are allowed to remain internalized permanently, physical problems manifest.

When the central nervous system and the cardiovascular system are stressed to constriction, major health problems occur over time. Doing Kelee meditation reverses the effects of stress by dissolving negative thought-form images in the mind, thus calming the central nervous system and the cardiovascular system at the same time.

As you practice Kelee meditation, mental strength and harmony of mind develop over time. It is harmony of mind that boosts the immune system and healing rates in the physical body.

> *Ron W. Rathbun*
> *Founder of Kelee Meditation*

The purest form of understanding occurs
when your mind
is not distracted by outside influences.
The deepest realizations
you will have in your life
will happen when you are alone
with your own thoughts.

Understanding the Difference Between Concentration and Meditation

To bring a sense of continuity to education of the mind, there must be an understanding everyone can agree upon in respect to concentration and meditation.

Concentration defined: The ability to focus without distraction, an active *doing* process.

Concentration is very important if you are to focus without distractions. No distractions, is an integral part of a high functioning mind. Without the ability to concentrate, mistakes are often made in relationship to what you are trying to achieve. Concentration is when you focus on a second point. All other mental disciplines that involve the process of doing something are in actuality concentration.

Meditation defined: A mind being still of thought, an awareness of nothing, an inactive *being* process.

A still mind is a mind at one point without an awareness of a second point. Attaining a still mind is the most difficult thing you can do and the most beneficial at the same time. An awareness of nothing is not an oxymoron; it is a mind with an awareness of nothing as a second point. This state of mind is called one-pointed stillness of mind and the goal and discipline of Kelee meditation.

Basic Principles of the Kelee Defined

1. Conscious Awareness: a point of perception between the intellectual outside physical world and your inside world of emotion.

2. Brain Function: thinks, analyzes, stores intellectual knowledge, and runs the physical body.

3. Mind Function: mentally feels or senses as an objective observer and is synonymous with a relaxed sense of perception; thus mind function leads into deeper states of awareness and innate knowing.

4. Surface of the Mind: a horizontal plane of electrochemical energy at eye level. A division point between the brain (or intellect) and deeper states of mind. These states are associated with inner contentment and an overall sense of calm.

5. Lesser Kelee: an electrochemical field of energy above the surface of the mind that moves out laterally from the center, up over the top of the brain, then down in between both hemispheres of the brain, and folds into the brain network. The energy in the lesser Kelee has to do with how you relate to the outside physical world—people, places, and things.

6. Greater Kelee: an electrochemical field of energy that flows below the surface of the mind, down to about where your heart is and then turns upward to join the lesser Kelee at the surface of the mind. The energy in the greater Kelee has to do with how you feel about yourself on an emotional level.

7. Compartments: synonymous with "baggage," emotional "buttons," or "issues" manifesting as nonproductive, inefficient behavioral traits.

8. Looping: occurs when your conscious awareness is attached to a negative compartment, resulting in a repetitive circulation of destructive thoughts.

9. Cessation of Looping: occurs when you are able to move your conscious awareness out of repetitive thinking into the open clear perception of mind.

10. Detachment from Internal Compartments: the space within your Kelee, where you live when you are unaffected by negative thoughts and emotions.

11. Processing of Compartments: the means by which internalized electrochemical negativity dissipates and dissolves. A result of relaxing your conscious awareness, stilling your mind, and detaching from compartments.

12. Flow of the Kelee: when the electrochemical energy of how you think and the energy of how you feel flow together in unison without beginning or end. The flow of the Kelee is realized by a single point of perception known as the conscious awareness.

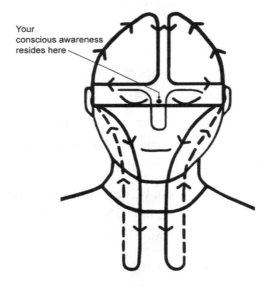

Your conscious awareness resides here

Chapter One

Conscious Awareness

Your conscious awareness

is a point of perception

between

the thinking intellectual process

associated with

the outside physical world

and your inside world

of feelings and

the abstraction of emotions.

Conscious Awareness

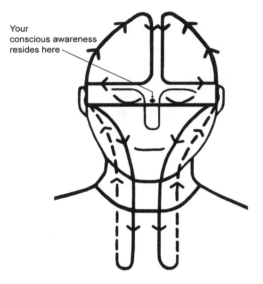

Your
conscious awareness
resides here

1. Your conscious awareness is who is reading this sentence right now. Your conscious awareness defines your relationship with yourself and the world around you.

Conscious Awareness

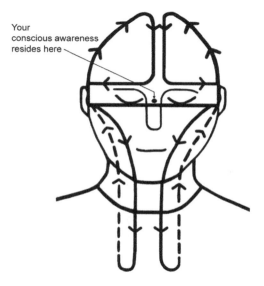

Your conscious awareness resides here

2. Your conscious awareness resides primarily at the surface of your mind, at eye level. However, it can move around on the surface of the mind. It can be directed at will to the front, either side, or the back of the surface of the mind. Your conscious awareness can also move into the lesser and greater Kelee.

Conscious Awareness

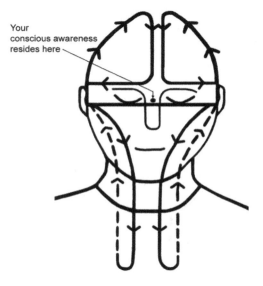

Your
conscious awareness
resides here

3. Your conscious awareness is the liaison between the intellectual outside physical world and your inside world of emotion. Your conscious awareness can move between brain and mind on command with training.

Conscious Awareness

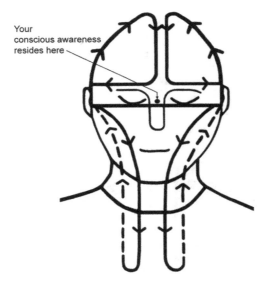

Your conscious awareness resides here

4. Where you direct your attention is where your conscious awareness will focus. What you focus on is called the secondary point. Where your conscious awareness perceives from in mind is called the primary point.

Conscious Awareness

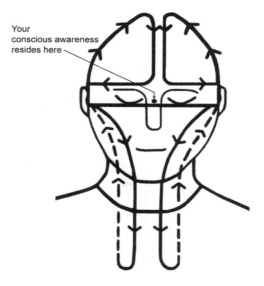

Your
conscious awareness
resides here

5. Your conscious awareness can be directed outward, into the outer physical environment to heighten awareness of physical surroundings (i.e., sights, sounds, movement).

Conscious Awareness

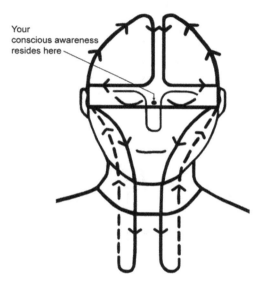

6. Your conscious awareness can be directed inward, so that you become self-aware of your inner world (i.e., thoughts, internalized fears, emotions).

Conscious Awareness

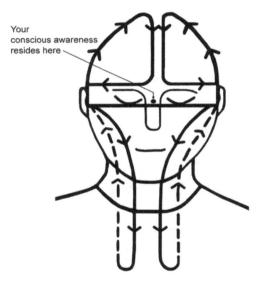

Your
conscious awareness
resides here

7. Your conscious awareness operates in three basic ways: mind function, brain function, and/or dysfunction (i.e., compartments).

Conscious Awareness

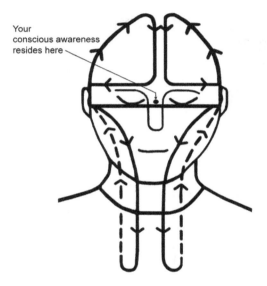

Your
conscious awareness
resides here

7a. Mind function: associated with your mental feeling sense or the observing part of you known as perception. This is your primary point.

Conscious Awareness

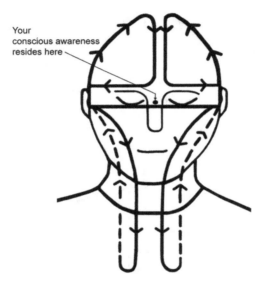

7b. Brain function: associated with the two physical hemispheres of your brain and your intellect. Your conscious awareness can be directed into your brain/intellect to think (i.e., read, spell, perform mathematical equations, or analyze concepts) in the lesser Kelee region.

Conscious Awareness

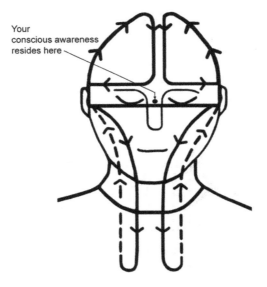

7c. Dysfunction: associated with misperception from compartments or negative "issues" (i.e., "baggage" or emotional "buttons") that are trapped in your Kelee.

Conscious Awareness

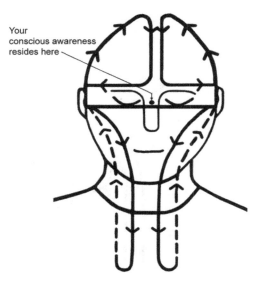

Your
conscious awareness
resides here

8. A truly conscious mind is continually learning and deepening in its understanding of subconscious and unconscious states of mind.

Conscious Awareness

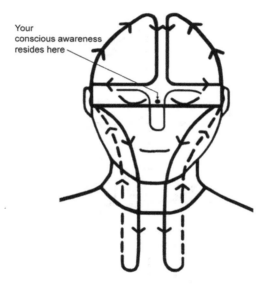

Your conscious awareness resides here

9. Conscious, subconscious, and unconscious are not separate states of mind. They are degrees of awareness.

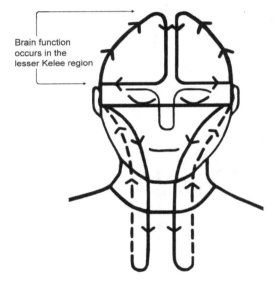

Brain function
occurs in the
lesser Kelee region

Chapter Two
Brain Function

Brain function
thinks, analyzes, stores
intellectual knowledge,
and runs the physical body.

Brain Function

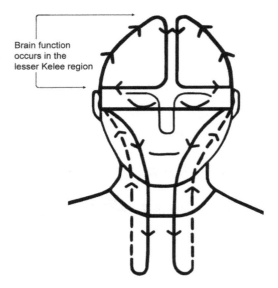

Brain function
occurs in the
lesser Kelee region

1. Brain function thinks, analyzes, stores data in the memory from existing knowledge in the intellect, runs the physical body, and is associated with the lesser Kelee region.

Brain Function

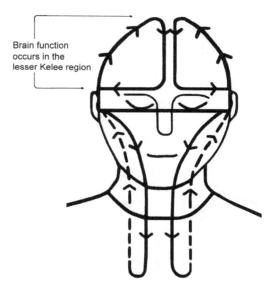

Brain function
occurs in the
lesser Kelee region

2. Brain function is associated with electrochemical physical energy. It is fueled by food energy on a physical level and fueled by the mind on a deeper more subtle level often called inspiration.

Brain Function

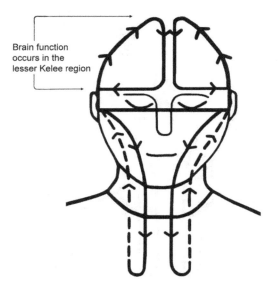

Brain function occurs in the lesser Kelee region

3. Look at the brain as an elaborate organic computer, it only does what you (i.e., the user) tell it to do.

Brain Function

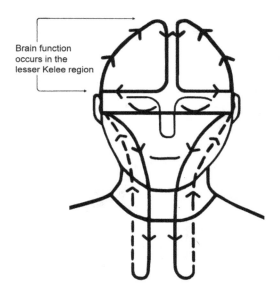

Brain function
occurs in the
lesser Kelee region

4. The brain works well when calm, while becoming fragmented when stressed.

Brain Function

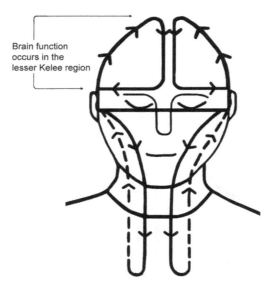

Brain function
occurs in the
lesser Kelee region

5. The tendency in brain function is to rationalize, justify, defend, and control how life is experienced. The brain operates in the three dimensions of height, width, and depth. It functions in association with the five physical senses and intellectualization.

Brain Function

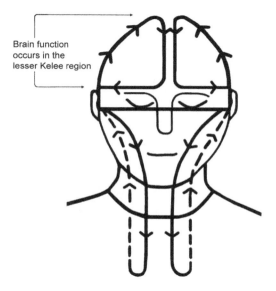

Brain function
occurs in the
lesser Kelee region

6. When you are unable to mentally feel a relaxed conscious awareness, you will remain thinking in brain function. You must be able to relax the brain to access clarity of mind.

Brain Function

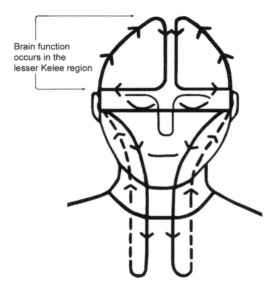

Brain function
occurs in the
lesser Kelee region

7. You must be able to locate and mentally feel your conscious awareness and allow it to relax and soften to begin the process of moving from brain function into mind function.

Brain Function

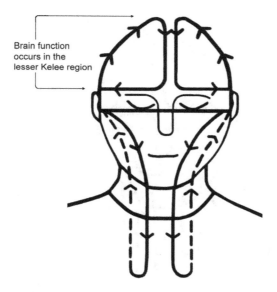

Brain function
occurs in the
lesser Kelee region

8. If you are not able to let go of the thinking or chatter from brain function, you will not enter into the calm, centered, deeper states of awareness experienced in mind function.

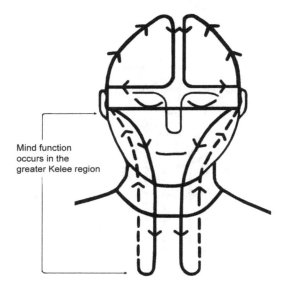

Mind function
occurs in the
greater Kelee region

Chapter Three

Mind Function

Mind function
mentally feels or senses
as an objective observer
and is synonymous with
a relaxed sense of perception;
thus mind function leads into
deeper states of awareness
and innate knowing.

Mind Function

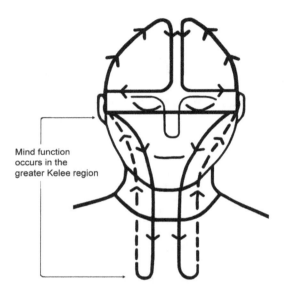

Mind function
occurs in the
greater Kelee region

1. Mind function mentally feels or senses as an objective observer and is synonymous with a relaxed feeling sense or clear perception.

Mind Function

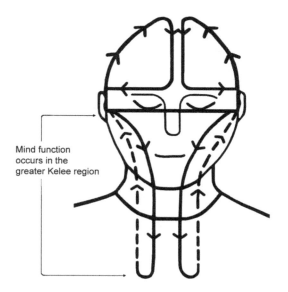

Mind function
occurs in the
greater Kelee region

2. This perception can extend beyond the three-dimensional experience into what can be loosely called intuition—a gut feeling, a hunch, or a vision that comes about. At the deepest level, it is seeing with absolute knowing.

Mind Function

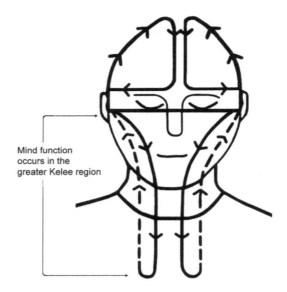

Mind function
occurs in the
greater Kelee region

3. Mind function leads into deeper states of awareness and knowing associated with the greater Kelee region. Knowing occurs when your mind senses with pure perception.

Mind Function

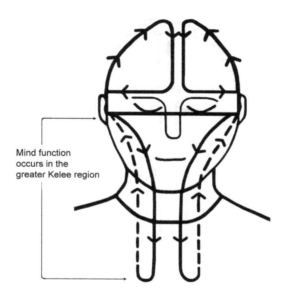

Mind function
occurs in the
greater Kelee region

4. Mind function is a relaxed, fluid, subtle form of energy. The mind is sentience—consciousness. It is considered an energy of the universe; it permeates every cell of the body. The depth of its understanding moves into vibratory states of awareness. The mind's awareness allows you to sense into unseen states of reality.

Mind Function

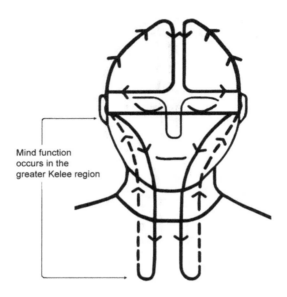

Mind function
occurs in the
greater Kelee region

5. The mind is our primary point of perception. Everything outside of primary point is called secondary point. When more energy is in second point than first point, we lose the mind's perception and default to brain function.

Mind Function

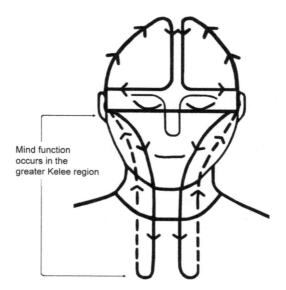

Mind function
occurs in the
greater Kelee region

6. To master mind function, you must let go of the thinking in brain function and allow your conscious awareness to drop inside, below the surface of the mind, and open up to your innate feeling sense found in the greater Kelee.

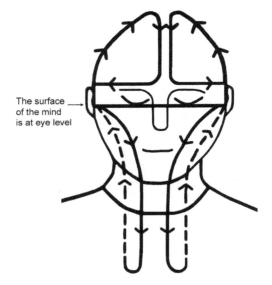

The surface of the mind is at eye level

Chapter Four

Surface of the Mind

*The surface of the mind
is a horizontal plane
of electrochemical energy
at eye level.
It is a reference point
to find your
conscious awareness
at any given moment.*

Surface of the Mind

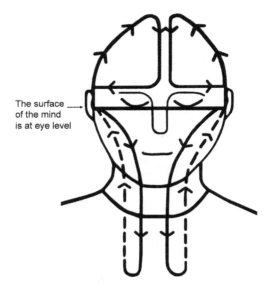

The surface ⟶ of the mind is at eye level

1. The surface of the mind is a flat plane of electrochemical energy at eye level. The surface of the mind literally splits between the pupils of the eyes. With practice, you can sense this.

Surface of the Mind

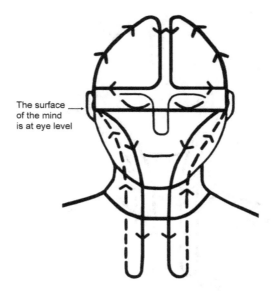

The surface
of the mind
is at eye level

2. The surface of the mind is a division point between the lesser Kelee and the greater Kelee. The lesser Kelee is associated with the brain and the intellect. The greater Kelee is associated with deeper states of mind and emotion.

Surface of the Mind

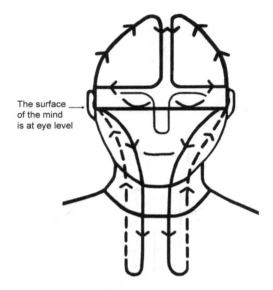

The surface of the mind is at eye level

3. Mentally feel where your thoughts are right now. You will feel them at eye level on the surface of the mind. It is the place the conscious awareness operates most often.

Surface of the Mind

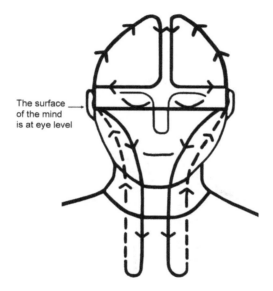

The surface
of the mind
is at eye level

4. The surface of the mind serves as a reception point for incoming information, a point of contemplation, and a place to make decisions. It is a horizon that links our brain function with the limitless space within us known as sentience—mind function.

Surface of the Mind

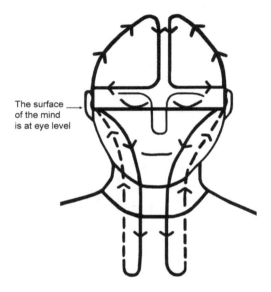

The surface of the mind is at eye level

5. Thinking takes place on the surface of the mind. It is also called the worktable of the mind. It is helpful to be aware of what is on the surface of the mind at all times. When things weigh on your mind, it is on the surface of the mind that you experience the weight.

Surface of the Mind

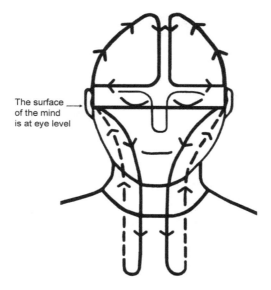

The surface
of the mind
is at eye level

6. The surface of the mind works best when cleared daily of distracting thoughts. A clean workspace invites our conscious awareness to work freely and in a more focused manner.

Surface of the Mind

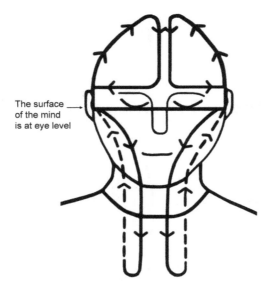

The surface
of the mind
is at eye level

7. Unresolved thoughts left on the surface of the mind tend to make you overthink things. Too many thoughts on the surface of the mind generate frustration, distraction, and fragmentation, thus potentially leading to the inability to focus.

Surface of the Mind

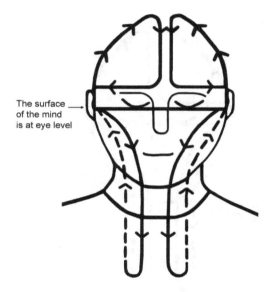

The surface of the mind is at eye level

8. When your conscious awareness is calm, relaxed, and centered on the surface of the mind you can focus on one thing. A natural effortless point of focus occurs when your conscious awareness is in mind function.

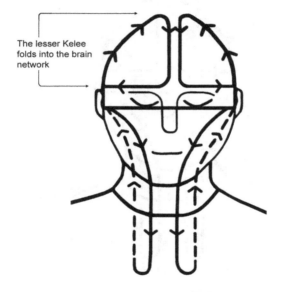

The lesser Kelee
folds into the brain
network

Chapter Five

Lesser Kelee

The lesser Kelee is an
electrochemical field of energy
above the surface of the mind
that moves out laterally
from the center,
up and over
the top of the brain,
then down in between
both hemispheres of the brain,
and then folds into
the brain network.

Lesser Kelee

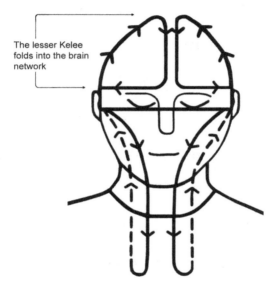

The lesser Kelee
folds into the brain
network

1. The energy of the lesser Kelee flows from the surface of the mind out laterally from the center, up and over the top of the brain, then down in between both hemispheres of the brain, and then folds into the brain network.

Lesser Kelee

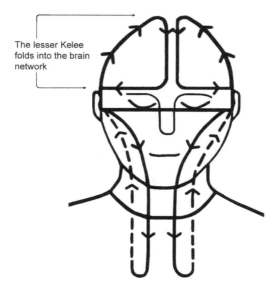

The lesser Kelee
folds into the brain
network

2. The lesser Kelee region is associated with the brain, the intellect, and the thinking process. It is also where the physical memory is located. An important part of everyday life is to not be forgetful by means of being in mind at one point (i.e., mind function).

Lesser Kelee

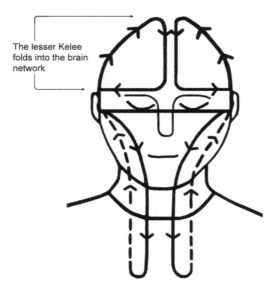

The lesser Kelee folds into the brain network

3. The lesser Kelee region is analytical, based in linear time, and operates in a three-dimensional realm of height, width, and depth.

Lesser Kelee

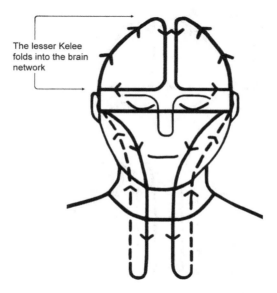

The lesser Kelee folds into the brain network

4. The lesser Kelee is the place where the mind can operate in close proximity to the brain. The long-term goal of Kelee meditation is to operate in mind whether in the lesser or greater Kelee.

Lesser Kelee

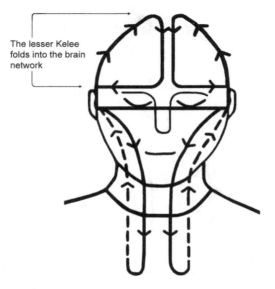

The lesser Kelee folds into the brain network

5. The lesser Kelee is where we can experience the space between our thoughts without interference from brain function. The space between our thoughts is the essence of the Kelee. The essence of the Kelee is our mind at the deepest level.

Lesser Kelee

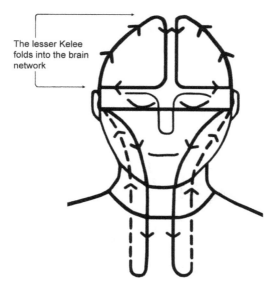

The lesser Kelee folds into the brain network

6. Compartments in the lesser Kelee region have to do with issues regarding the outside physical world—people, places, and things.

Lesser Kelee

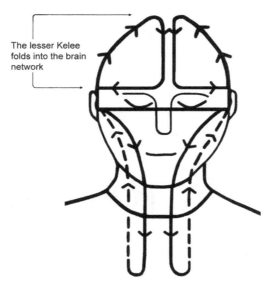

The lesser Kelee folds into the brain network

7. The most physically uncomfortable compartments in the lesser Kelee region are tension-based headaches, which are formed when you have either accepted or created negative experiences.

Lesser Kelee

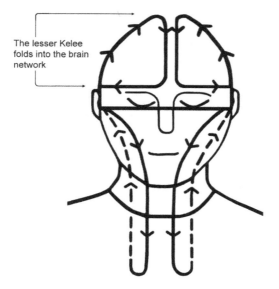

The lesser Kelee
folds into the brain
network

8. Your conscious awareness, associated with the lesser Kelee region, tends to create attachments to people and things in an attempt to be in control. Attachments are the root of all suffering in the human condition—with detachment being the means by which one finds freedom from suffering.

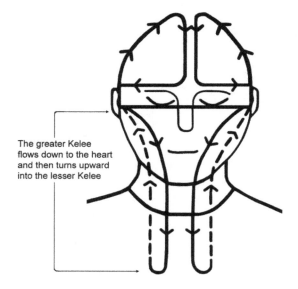

The greater Kelee
flows down to the heart
and then turns upward
into the lesser Kelee

Chapter Six

Greater Kelee

*T*he greater Kelee is an
electrochemical field of energy
that flows
below the surface of the mind,
down to about
where your heart is
and then turns upward
to join the lesser Kelee
at the surface of the mind.

Greater Kelee

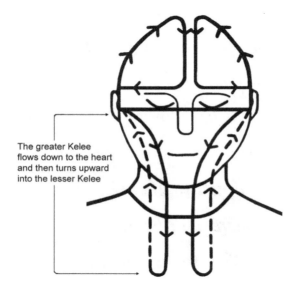

The greater Kelee flows down to the heart and then turns upward into the lesser Kelee

1. The energy of the greater Kelee flows from the surface of the mind, down to about where your heart is and then turns upward to join in with the lesser Kelee. The greater and the lesser Kelee are actually one Kelee folding in upon each other connected by our conscious awareness.

Greater Kelee

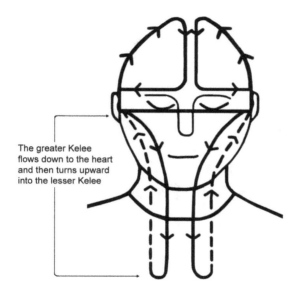

The greater Kelee flows down to the heart and then turns upward into the lesser Kelee

2. The greater Kelee is associated with a feeling process, emotion, and matters of the heart. It is also where you can enter into mind without the distraction that can come from brain function.

Greater Kelee

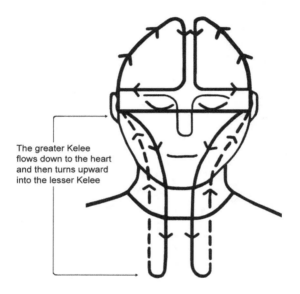

The greater Kelee
flows down to the heart
and then turns upward
into the lesser Kelee

3. The greater Kelee is non-linear in nature and operates without an awareness of time. Because there is no physical matter in the greater Kelee, there is no matter moving through space, which defines time. In mind, time stands still because there is none. Mind is where perception and patience occur naturally.

Greater Kelee

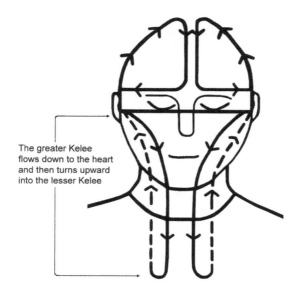

The greater Kelee
flows down to the heart
and then turns upward
into the lesser Kelee

4. The greater Kelee is infinite in nature. If you are to perceive the infinite, you cannot use mass as your measuring point, such is the nature of the greater Kelee and that of the mind.

Greater Kelee

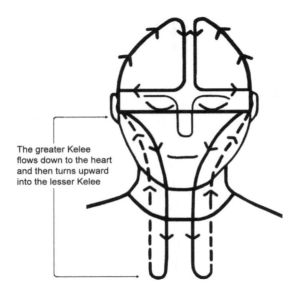

The greater Kelee
flows down to the heart
and then turns upward
into the lesser Kelee

5. The greater Kelee is where you can move out of analytical thinking, and with practice, move into pure perception of mind.

Greater Kelee

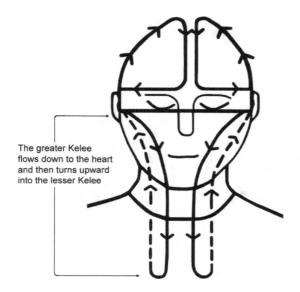

The greater Kelee
flows down to the heart
and then turns upward
into the lesser Kelee

6. The greater Kelee is where emotion (i.e., abstract sensation) flows from as an expression of you. The need to express emotion is at the heart of human nature. Without this drive, we would not evolve, which is mankind's eternal quest.

Greater Kelee

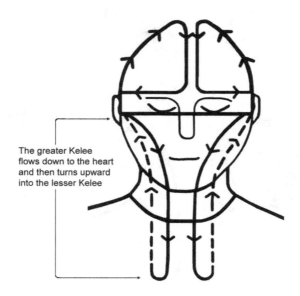

The greater Kelee flows down to the heart and then turns upward into the lesser Kelee

7. The greater Kelee is a vessel of electrochemical energy that contains your "heart" and emotion (i.e., abstract sensation).

Greater Kelee

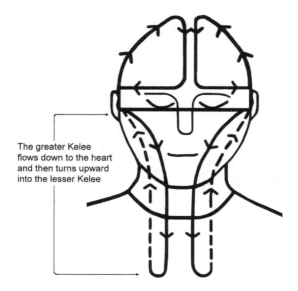

The greater Kelee
flows down to the heart
and then turns upward
into the lesser Kelee

8. To understand this abstract sensation known as emotion, you must learn to mentally feel with your mind. This allows you to accurately perceive what emotion is, without using a preconceived intellectual understanding of that emotion. Only then will you begin to experience the deeper realms of abstract sensation (i.e., emotion).

Greater Kelee

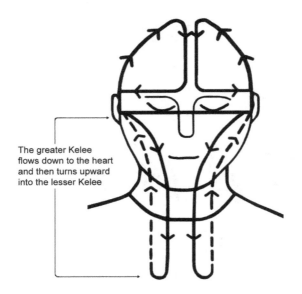

The greater Kelee
flows down to the heart
and then turns upward
into the lesser Kelee

9. Defining how you feel will evolve when you understand that you can physically feel and you can mentally feel. When you can mentally feel, you will open your perception to unrealized states of mind that you will have to experience for yourself.

Greater Kelee

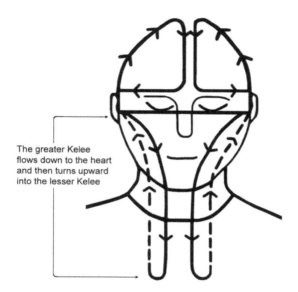

The greater Kelee flows down to the heart and then turns upward into the lesser Kelee

10. The emotion of a heartache is the hardest of all human experiences. It is solved not by using the brain, but by using the mind to understand that two people can never be as one. However, two people can touch softly with beautiful emotion from one to another.

Greater Kelee

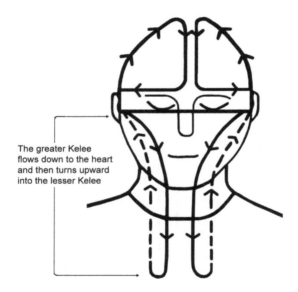

The greater Kelee flows down to the heart and then turns upward into the lesser Kelee

11. Everyone at one time or another has felt emotion well up from within the greater Kelee. When you can learn to mentally feel mind function on command, you can begin to explore the greater Kelee and the deeper realms of emotion.

Greater Kelee

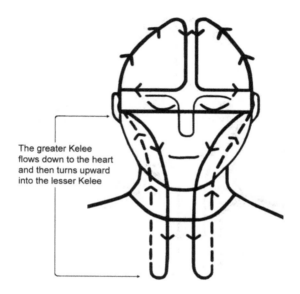

The greater Kelee
flows down to the heart
and then turns upward
into the lesser Kelee

12. To access mind function, you must learn how to switch your focus from the brain and the lesser Kelee region and allow your conscious awareness to drop into the greater Kelee, where you begin to enter deeper states of mind.

Greater Kelee

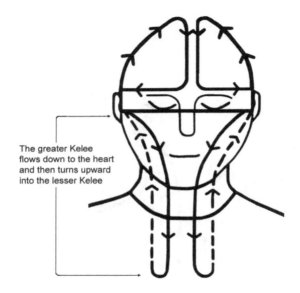

The greater Kelee
flows down to the heart
and then turns upward
into the lesser Kelee

13. The greater Kelee is where you can learn to be completely still at one point. Complete stillness of mind at its deepest level is an awareness of nothing. When a second point does not exist, there can be nothing to distract you. One-pointed stillness is the goal of Kelee meditation.

Greater Kelee

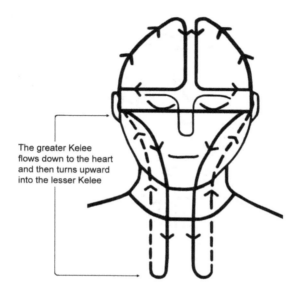

The greater Kelee
flows down to the heart
and then turns upward
into the lesser Kelee

14. The greater Kelee is where the emotions of love and contentment are realized and then experienced. When you open to the inspiration that comes from your greater Kelee, life feels good because you do. When you feel good, this leads to self-acceptance and your own beautiful self-acceptance leads to love.

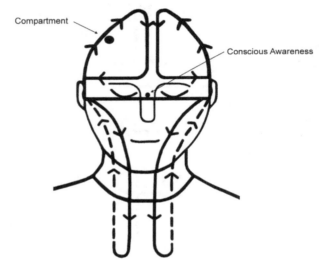

Compartment

Conscious Awareness

Chapter Seven

Compartments

Compartments
are synonymous with
"baggage," emotional "buttons,"
or "issues" manifesting as
nonproductive, inefficient
behavioral traits.

Compartments

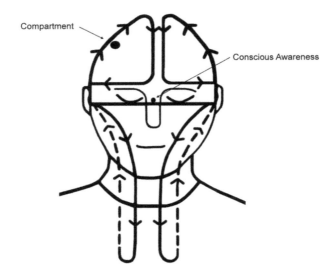

1. Compartments are called many names in our society: "baggage," "issues," emotional "buttons," and dysfunction, to name a few. Compartments appear in forms of boxes, stacks of paper, or images of people. Compartments can take the shape of almost any image that reminds you of a problem.

Compartments

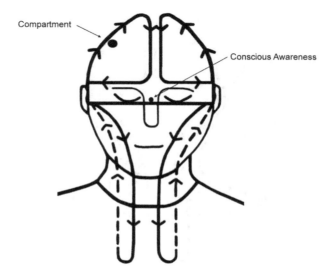

2. From birth until this moment in time, energy from life experience is pouring through your mind. When you, not knowing any better, take in a negative experience, the thought can become trapped in the Kelee as a compartment.

Compartments

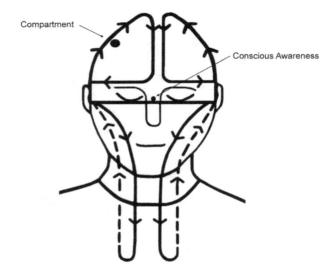

3. Your conscious awareness thinks and mentally perceives in thought-form images. Harmonious thought-form images go directly to memory and do not compartmentalize.

Compartments

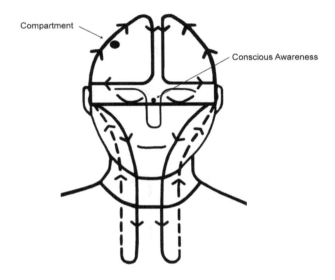

4. However, when disharmonious (i.e., negative) thought-form images enter your Kelee, they can become trapped as compartments when you cannot let them go.

Compartments

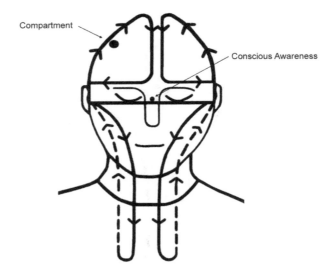

5. Compartments form in two basic ways—from an outside circumstance or we create them:

    a. When you internalize a negative experience in an effort to control negativity.

    b. When you cannot face the harshness of reality and internally self-create an illusion to offset discomfort.

Compartments

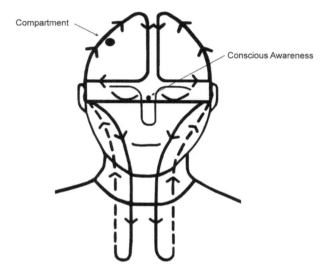

6. Compartments can form in three main areas:
   a. On the surface of the mind.
   b. In the lesser Kelee.
   c. In the greater Kelee.

Compartments

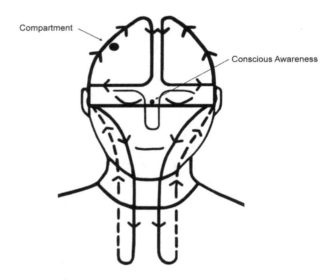

7. There are two extreme forms of compartments:
   a. Anxiety-based.
   b. Depression-based.
   Both drain electrochemical energy from the immune system.

Compartments

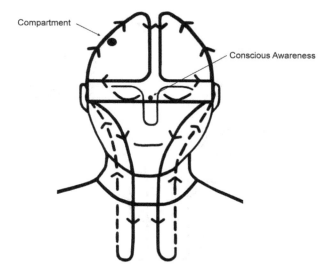

8. There are two basic ways compartments get energy and stay alive:

    a. By engaging your conscious awareness (e.g., being angry or adverserial with yourself).

    b. By engaging another (e.g., being angry or adverserial with another).

Compartments

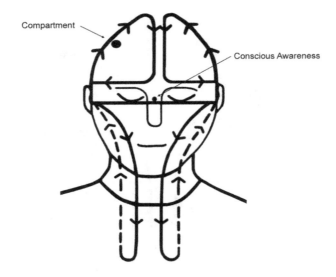

9. Compartments can exist in a conscious, subconscious, or unconscious form. Compartments are most often subconscious or unconscious because you do not want to look at them or you have become comfortable with being uncomfortable. Unfortunately, they can still affect you even if your behavior is unconscious to you.

Compartments

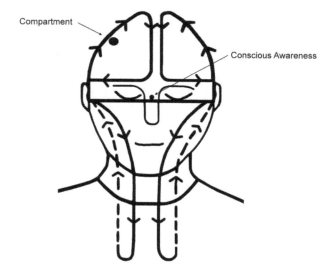

Compartments affect the conscious awareness in three ways:
10a. Being consumed: when your conscious awareness is consumed by a compartment, and you are completely controlled by it and unaware of how the compartment is influencing your behavior. This is when your behavior can be unconsciously and/or subconsciously driven.

Compartments

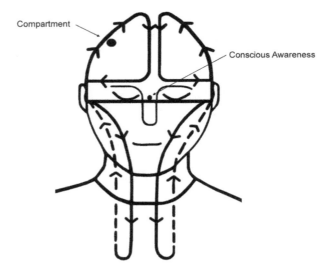

10b. Being influenced: when your conscious awareness feels the compartment, but you are not controlled by it and you are aware of the compartment's influence. This is when you are conscious of your behavior.

Compartments

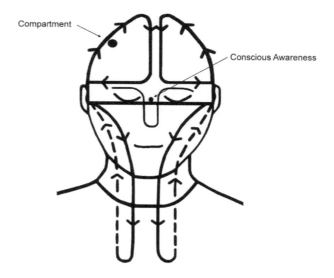

10c. Being free: when your conscious awareness is unaffected by compartments and you are totally aware of your freedom. Being free is also a state of mind known as detachment.

Compartments

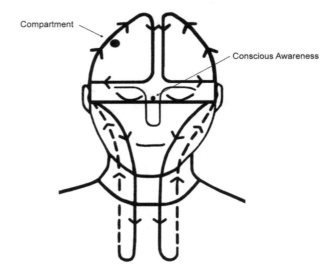

11. All compartments are controlled ways of being which do not allow us to grow mentally and become comfortable with change. When you can detach and stop thinking about them, freedom of mind occurs along with happiness and contentment.

Compartments

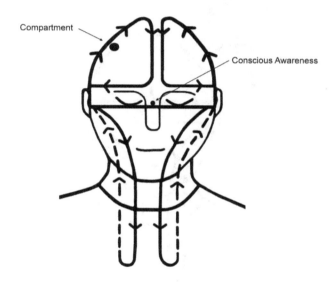

12. Compartments are mental blocks that hinder the learning process. Removal of mental blocks happens by means of processing and dissolving compartments. When compartments are dissolved, learning flourishes.

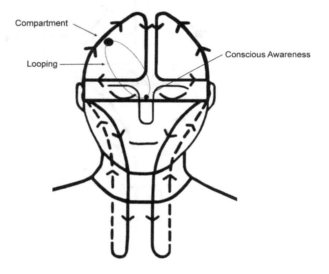

Chapter Eight
Looping

*Looping occurs when
your conscious awareness
is attached to
a negative compartment
resulting in a repetitive circulation
of hurtful thoughts.*

Looping

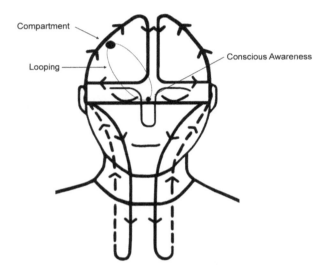

1. When your conscious awareness attaches to a negative compartment it can repeatedly circulate through the negativity, in a closed loop without resolution. This is when looping occurs.

Looping

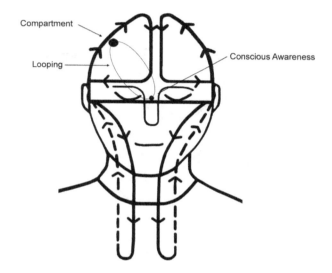

2. Unresolved repetitive thoughts occur when you do not understand something about yourself, others, or the world at large. Unresolved thoughts are not weakness, but an opportunity from which to learn. Awareness that you are looping is the first step to ending it.

Looping

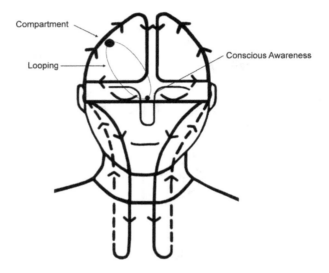

3. When a compartment is triggered by external stimuli, your conscious awareness can react by trying to control what is triggering you. When you try to control a compartment, you become part of the loop. When you can relax your conscious awareness into primary point of mind, looping dissipates and the compartment can begin processing out.

Looping

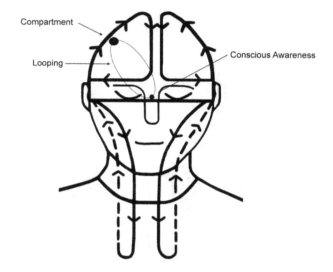

4. A closed loop of disappointment between your conscious awareness and a compartment will result in a constant stream of negative chattering thoughts. When you are chattering and looping, it is because you have temporarily "lost your mind" and have been consumed by a compartment that wants to control your conscious awareness. Remember, when you are in primary point of mind, you do not chatter and loop.

Looping

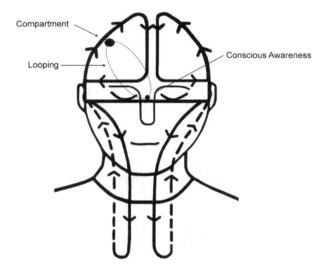

5. Being aware that you are looping is the first step to ending it. Looping happens when your conscious awareness, from the intellect, cannot stop thinking about something or someone. When you relax into mind function, you move into a subtle form of energy in the mind that does not loop, it perceives.

Looping

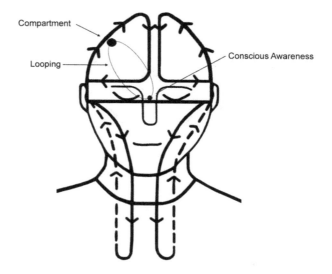

6. You loop because you are looking for resolution in a place that does not have it—your memory—from the intellect. Trying to understand something new, in the present, from incomplete information from the past, causes looping. This looping occurs when the conscious awareness searches a past event for resolution that is not there, but still continues to search.

Looping

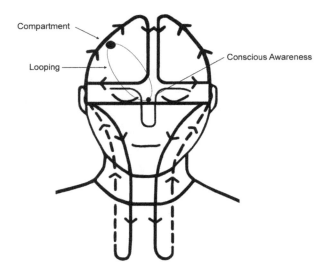

7. Looping keeps you trapped in the past because all compartments are rooted in previous disharmonious experiences. This interferes with living openly to experience life in the present moment. Everything in the past is based in second point. If you are to truly live and be in the present, you must be in primary point of mind.

Looping

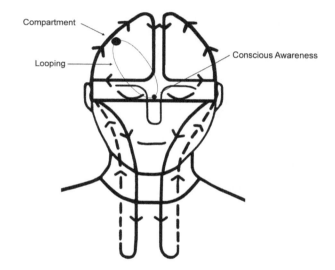

8. You can loop with your own compartments or with another person's compartments. It is from doing something that you loop. It is from doing nothing that you do not. If you are to learn to stop looping, you must learn to observe without doing, in primary point of mind.

Looping

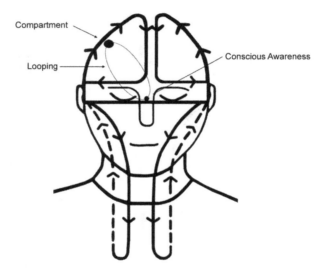

9. When your conscious awareness has more energy in a second point (i.e., compartment) and you cannot stop thinking about the second point from brain function, you will loop. Remember, the energy of mind does not loop, it flows.

Looping

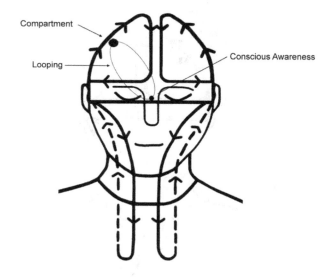

10. An object of your attention—the second point—cannot understand itself for you. You may see the object of attention at the second point, but without your perception of mind in the primary point, you see but do not understand. It is like reading a page but not understanding what you read. Learn to read life with your mind and you will end looping.

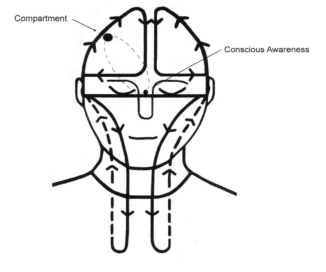

Chapter Nine
Cessation of Looping

*Cessation of looping occurs
when you are able to move
your conscious awareness
out of repetitive thinking
into the clear perception of mind.*

Cessation of Looping

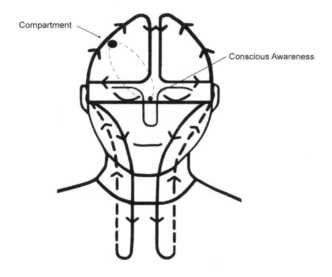

1. When you are able to move your conscious awareness out of repetitive thinking into the clear perception of mind, the cycle of looping is broken.

Cessation of Looping

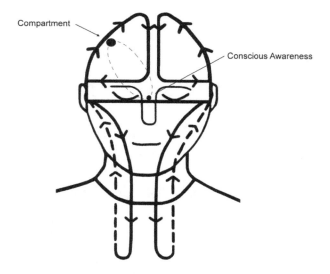

2. Looping ends when perception of mind begins. Looping is a two-point process and perception of mind is a one-point process, therefore looping does not occur in mind function. The energy of mind coexists in the physical world, but is not based in it. There is an energy in the universe and that same energy is the energy of mind.

Cessation of Looping

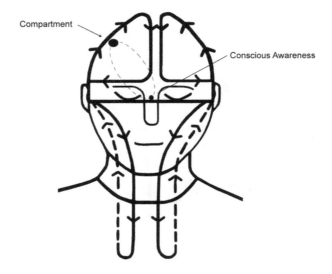

3. The first step to stop looping is to know that it is occurring and to stop thinking. The key is to mentally locate the energy of your conscious awareness and calm it by allowing it to relax and soften. Calming the energy of your conscious awareness is how you move from brain function into mind function.

Cessation of Looping

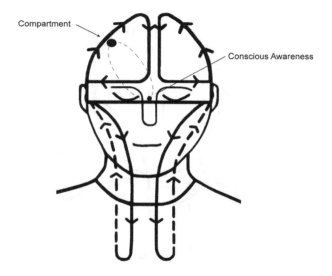

4. Looping is diminished when you consciously calm the electrochemical energy of brain function. When the energy of brain function escalates, looping is fueled. It is the calm energy of mind function that weakens looping and ultimately breaks the cycle. When looping is broken, the associated compartments are not fueled, thus isolating compartments to consume their own fuel until they dissipate.

Cessation of Looping

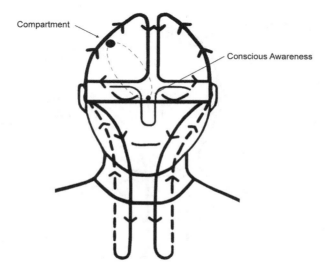

5. Looping is further diminished when your conscious awareness relaxes and does not engage with your compartments or another person's compartments.

Cessation of Looping

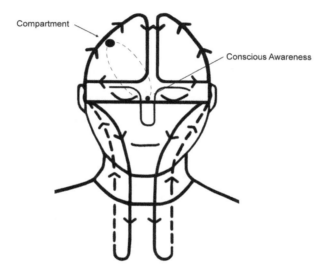

6. Looping is broken when you learn to live *detached in mind function* instead of *attached in brain function.* Detachment is learned through doing Kelee meditation.

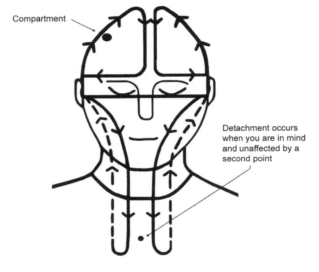

Compartment

Detachment occurs
when you are in mind
and unaffected by a
second point

Chapter Ten

Detachment from Internal Compartments

Detachment

from internal compartments

is found

in the open space

within your Kelee,

where you live

when you are unaffected by

negative thoughts and emotions.

Detachment from Internal Compartments

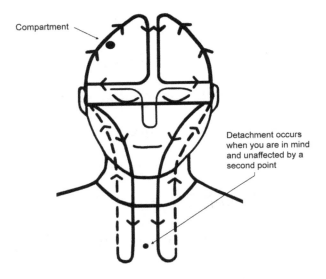

Compartment

Detachment occurs when you are in mind and unaffected by a second point

1. Detachment refers to the state of being (versus doing), when you are unaffected by negative emotion. It is also a state of freedom where perception is learned. Detachment from a second point is experienced when you are in primary point of mind.

Detachment from Internal Compartments

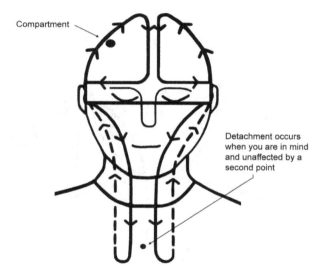

2. When you mentally attach to people or things, a dependency is formed. When the attachment is broken, this leads to emotional and/or physical pain (e.g., a compartment).

Detachment from Internal Compartments

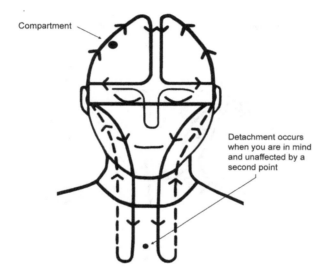

Compartment

Detachment occurs when you are in mind and unaffected by a second point

3. Detachment defines a truly open mind. It allows you to live freely by seeing life as it really is—not how the influence of the outside world (e.g., family, friends, socialization) would have you see life.

Detachment from Internal Compartments

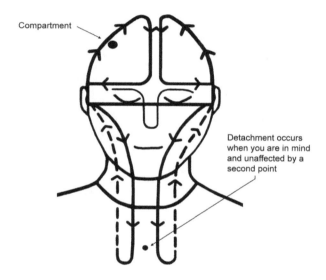

Compartment

Detachment occurs
when you are in mind
and unaffected by a
second point

4. People form attachments as a way of trying to control people, places, or things either directly or indirectly. It is said, "The ultimate form of control is to not control at all." When you allow life to be, it allows you to be—yourself.

Detachment from Internal Compartments

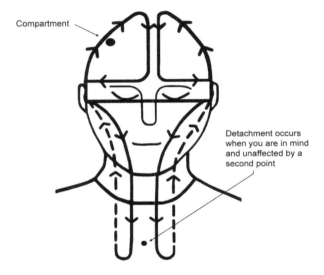

Compartment

Detachment occurs
when you are in mind
and unaffected by a
second point

5. When you try to mentally control another—interference occurs. When interference occurs, disharmony is the result. The way to end interference is to start the practice of non-interference. This non-interference occurs from detachment learned in primary point of mind.

Detachment from Internal Compartments

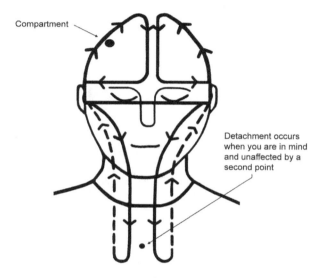

Compartment

Detachment occurs
when you are in mind
and unaffected by a
second point

6. To learn detachment, you must learn to be still at one
point in mind. When you are still at one point, you cannot be
attached to a second point at the same time.

Detachment from Internal Compartments

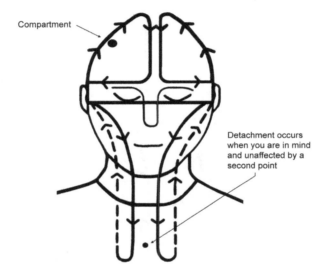

Compartment

Detachment occurs
when you are in mind
and unaffected by a
second point

7. At the deepest level, detachment is learned when you can drop your conscious awareness into your greater Kelee and be still and unaffected by any thoughts. It is by practicing one-pointed stillness that you learn to live in mind, and thus, live detached from what affects you.

Detachment from Internal Compartments

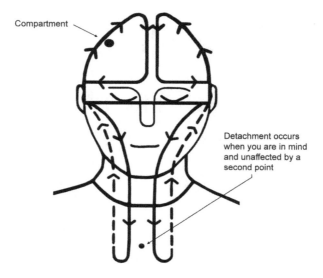

Compartment

Detachment occurs when you are in mind and unaffected by a second point

There are three basic steps to learn detachment:

8a. Mentally locate and feel the energy of your conscious awareness and allow it to soften and relax. Relaxing your conscious awareness through compartments in the lesser Kelee region dissolves them over time.

Detachment from Internal Compartments

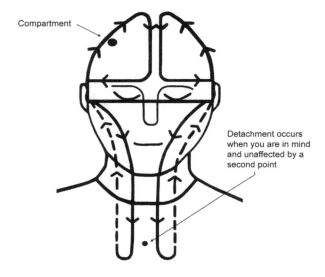

Compartment

Detachment occurs when you are in mind and unaffected by a second point

8b. Allow your relaxed conscious awareness to open to the innate space found in the greater Kelee, and learn to be still at one point.

Detachment from Internal Compartments

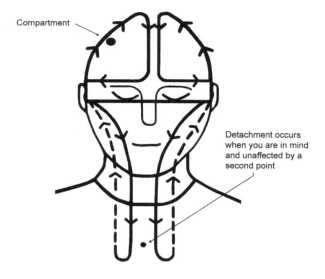

Compartment

Detachment occurs
when you are in mind
and unaffected by a
second point

8c. When your conscious awareness is detached from negative thoughts or emotions, you remove the energy source that keeps compartments alive. When you live in mind function, you will detach from compartments, and they will dissolve. When you detach from what *isn't* you, you find what *is* you.

Detachment from Internal Compartments

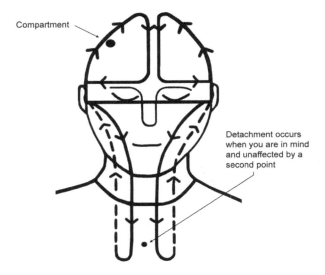

Compartment

Detachment occurs when you are in mind and unaffected by a second point

9. Detachment, in simple terms, is not being something other than who you are. What you are not, is your compartments or misperceptions of yourself. What you are, in your purest state is a conscious uninterrupted flow of life experience.

Detachment from Internal Compartments

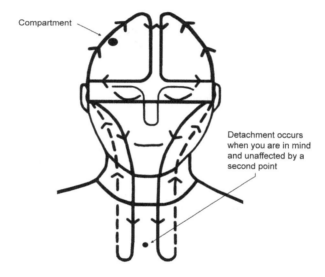

Compartment

Detachment occurs when you are in mind and unaffected by a second point

10. Detachment is not a self-created mental state of isolation or separation from others. Instead, detachment is a feeling of being connected to yourself and others, without the pain associated with attachment. Detachment in the purest sense is the absence of separation with all people, places, and things.

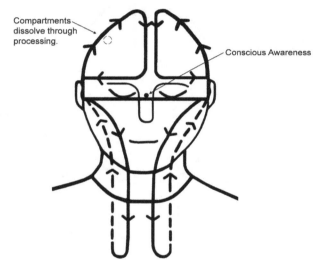

Compartments dissolve through processing.

Conscious Awareness

Chapter Eleven

Processing of Compartments

Processing of compartments
is how
internalized
electrochemical negativity
dissipates and dissolves.

Processing of Compartments

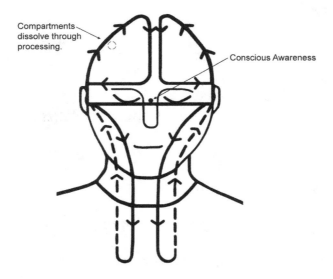

1. Processing internal negative compartments begins when your own mental resistance relaxes. Tension in your conscious awareness feeds compartments, whereas relaxation does not. Everything done when relaxed is easier, everything done while tense is harder.

Processing of Compartments

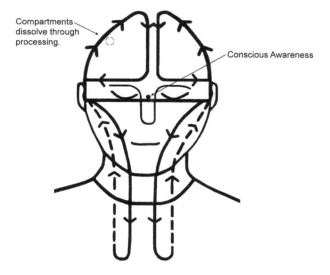

2. In order to avoid feeling the negativity of a compartment, most people block out "issues" by the self-creation of an electrochemical mental wall of resistance. In actuality, this technique reinforces and keeps compartments alive in your Kelee. It is an illusion that you can permanently protect yourself from feeling your compartments. The only way to not feel your compartments is to dissolve them.

Processing of Compartments

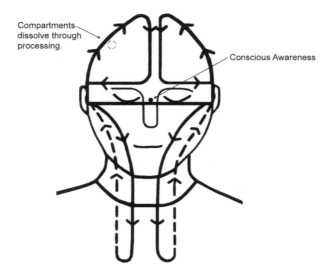

Compartments dissolve through processing.

Conscious Awareness

3. You may feel emotional discomfort or moodiness while processing; however, when the compartment dissolves, you will not experience the influence of that particular compartment again. When you have had a compartment your whole life and it is simply gone—this you will have to experience to believe.

Processing of Compartments

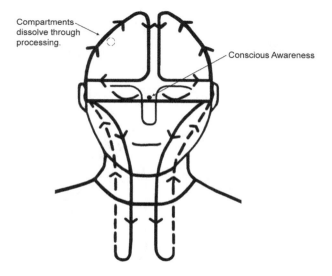

Compartments dissolve through processing.

Conscious Awareness

4. It's common to experience physiological effects when processing, such as low energy, headaches, nausea, depression, or anxiety. If a compartment was linked with physical discomfort at the time it formed, it will mimic the same response when it processes out. The physical discomfort will cease when the compartment is released.

Processing of Compartments

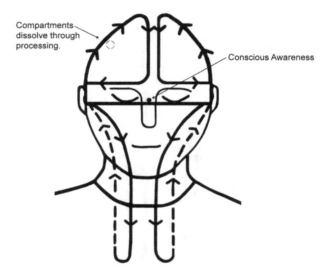

Compartments dissolve through processing.

Conscious Awareness

5. When a compartment dissolves, it cannot be triggered again. Some compartments can appear similar, but upon close inspection, they are not. You may have layers of similar types of compartments that are chronologically stacked in your Kelee.

Processing of Compartments

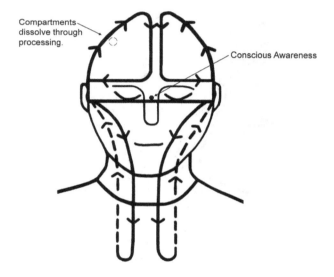

Compartments dissolve through processing.

Conscious Awareness

6. Processing is a classic sign that Kelee meditation is working correctly. You can either process or be moody. The physiological effects of processing tend to be short-term in duration, whereas being moody (associated with looping) can be long-term in duration. Processing is like having to take out the trash. It is an unpleasant thing to do, but necessary to remain clean.

Processing of Compartments

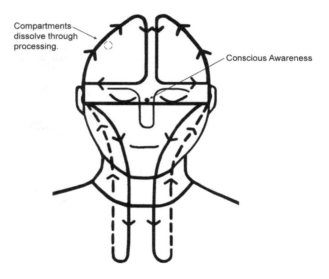

Compartments dissolve through processing.

Conscious Awareness

7. Processing allows compartments to burn their own electrochemical energy and not yours. Once compartments dissipate, you will not experience them again.

Processing of Compartments

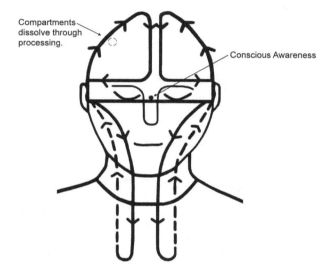

8. Ponder how many times a day that a compartment has been triggered over your lifetime. How much time each day has been consumed looping through these compartments? Now look at how much more time you will have without them. Time seems to appear out of nowhere when you are not distracted by compartments from your past.

Processing of Compartments

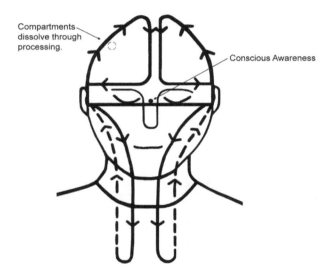

Compartments dissolve through processing.

Conscious Awareness

9. Understanding the basic principles of the Kelee and doing Kelee meditation provides you with a choice: You can loop endlessly through compartments and sustain them, or you can process your compartments until they dissolve.

Processing of Compartments

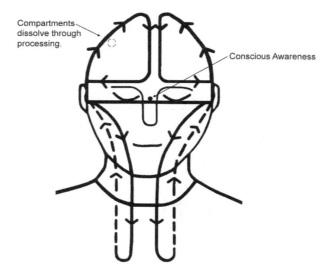

Compartments
dissolve through
processing.

Conscious Awareness

10. When you do Kelee meditation, the choice becomes clear—processing is better than looping. The harmonious feeling of having one less compartment after processing outweighs any physiological effects that may occur during processing.

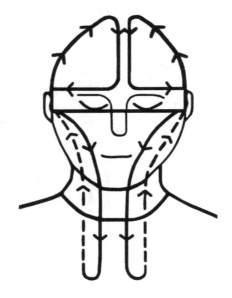

Chapter Twelve
Flow of the Kelee

The flow of the Kelee
is when
the electrochemical energy
of how you think
and the energy
of how you feel
flow together
without beginning or end
in perfect unison
with time.

Flow of the Kelee

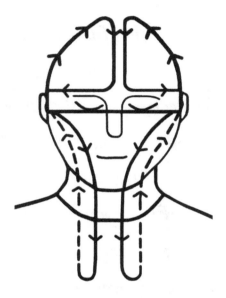

1. Within the Kelee, the three-dimensional linear moment of time meets the non-linear moment of mental feeling and perception. It is in bringing these two energies in harmony together at the surface of the mind that balance is achieved.

Flow of the Kelee

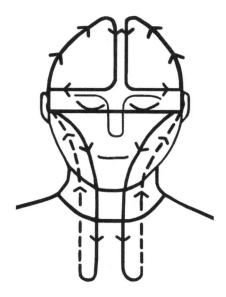

2. The energy of the Kelee flows in upon itself, without beginning or end. Within the flow of the Kelee is a single point of perception known as the conscious awareness. It is in understanding your conscious awareness that you begin to understand the subconscious and unconscious depths of your mind.

Flow of the Kelee

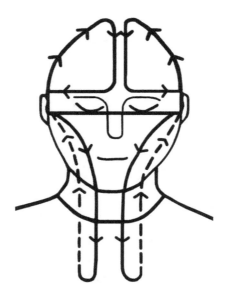

3. When you hear of the proverbial flow of life, this is when the energy of the lesser Kelee (what you think) and the energy of the greater Kelee (how you feel) flow together in harmony.

Flow of the Kelee

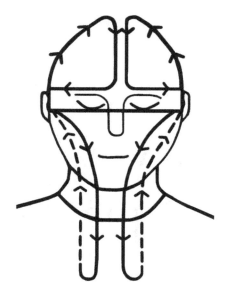

4. Everyone has a choice to either loop through the memory of who you think you are, or flow with who you feel you are, in this present moment. When you pay attention to your mind, you realize that you think what you don't know and feel what you do. Thinking is when you are looking for resolution. Mental feeling is when you are open to the acceptance of resolution.

Flow of the Kelee

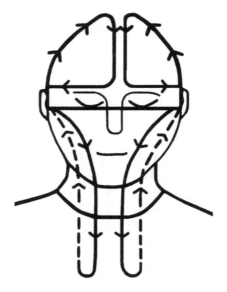

5. When you're centered in your conscious awareness, you can learn to flow with the harmonious energy of your Kelee. It is from feeling the flow of your Kelee that the eternal moment is realized, also known as "the now."

Flow of the Kelee

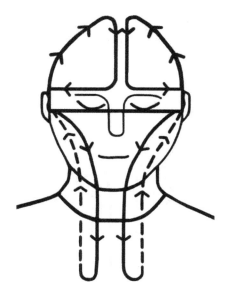

6. To open to the flow of the Kelee, you must learn how to end your own internal struggle between your negative self-image and the essence of who you really are. The struggle in your conscious awareness ends when relaxation starts in the mind. It is in letting go of control-based tension, that a relaxed sense of *being* in the mind is found.

Flow of the Kelee

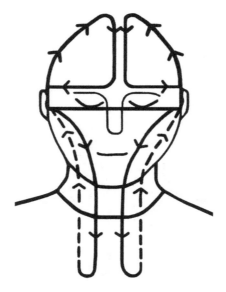

7. The essence of who you really are is found in your greater Kelee. The key to opening to the flow of the Kelee is in learning to calm your physical energy with the energy of mind. When your conscious awareness is at ease, you will naturally merge into the open space of mind.

Flow of the Kelee

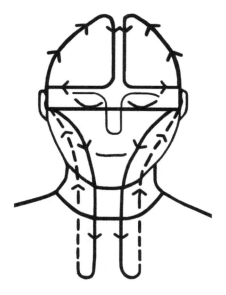

8. Calmness in the mind balances the physical. Stillness in the mind balances the mental. The vibratory range of energy from calmness to stillness is immense and will be understood through your study of the Kelee and that of one-pointed stillness.

Flow of the Kelee

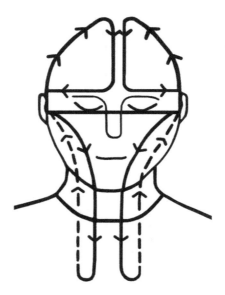

9. The flow of the Kelee is a model of the universe. It is infinitely large folding in upon itself without beginning or end, with only a point of perception to perceive from. Without perception from sentience, does the universe exist.

Flow of the Kelee

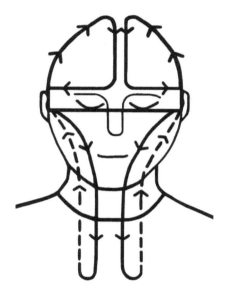

10. When your conscious awareness can perceive from the open space of mind instead of mass-based seeing, a new measurement of reality will be realized. It is in learning to move from the seen to the unseen that reverse mass is perceived. Reverse mass is a vibratory rate with non-physical structure, commonly known in the Kelee as compartments.

Flow of the Kelee

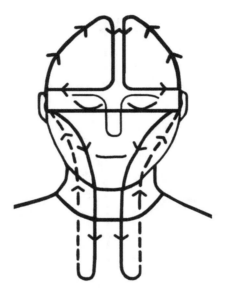

11. The Kelee flows in perfect sync with time. It allows time and space to cohabitate in perfect harmony, when you do not try to control time and space. It is in understanding non-linear time that you will learn how to perceive time and space in their unaltered state.

Flow of the Kelee

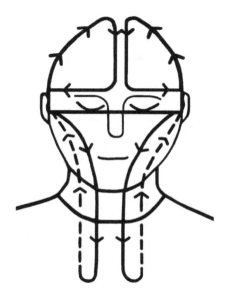

12. The Kelee opens you to *be*, yet allows you to *do*, with a free will. The Kelee is a vessel of energy. This vessel is a place where you can take bad things out and put good things in. What you do with your energy determines your mistakes or your successes. The choice is yours to use this knowledge or not.

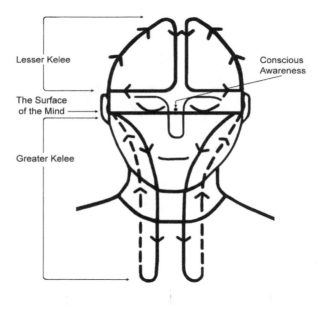

Lesser Kelee

Conscious Awareness

The Surface of the Mind

Greater Kelee

Chapter Thirteen
Overview of Kelee Meditation

The Kelee
brings new meaning
to the term
"internal" medicine.

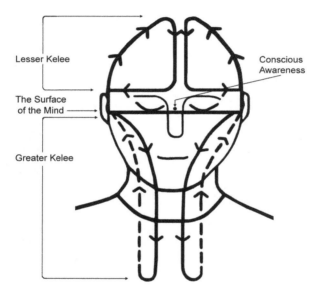

Overview of Kelee Meditation

Science itself relies mainly on the intellect of the brain to convey proof; however, when the intellect hits a wall, frustration usually sets in if the problem is not solved. When the problem goes on long enough, the researcher or physician starts to speculate about the possibilities. As speculation does not produce the answer, pondering starts and a line is crossed from speculating in brain function to pondering in mind function.

Pondering in primary point is a gentle form of mental observation in mind, which leads to letting go of presupposition from the brain. This is the start to perception in the mind. It took humanity quite some time to recognize that even though you cannot see germs with the human eye, they still exist—just like compartments.

As you begin to still the mind repetitively over a period of time, clarity of mind develops. Instead of learning only through established, secondhand intellectual knowledge from books or from others, you gain an additional ability of being open to experiencing deeper levels of firsthand knowledge and understanding.

In other words, you see and understand things that your mind is fascinated about firsthand for yourself—not from what you read or what others tell you about. This is true learning at its finest and where new, unseen discoveries come from—a still mind. Harmony produces the ability to see clearly and disharmony creates confusion, known as compartments.

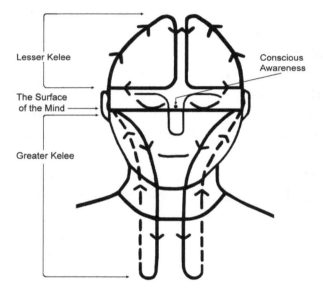

Overview of Kelee Meditation

Step One

Locate and mentally feel your conscious awareness at the top of the head. From the top of your head, mentally relax your conscious awareness into a flat plane of awareness. Allow this plane of awareness to soften and pass through both hemispheres of the brain, ultimately settling at the surface of the mind. When a thought or image distracts your conscious awareness, simply let it pass by. At the surface of the mind, you should be mentally calm and relaxed, but not actively thinking. When the relaxed horizontal plane of conscious awareness reaches the surface of the mind, gently bring your conscious awareness to a single point of perception. Step One should take about two minutes.

Step Two

From a single point of perception, allow your conscious awareness to drop below the surface of the mind to a natural still point within your greater Kelee. Letting go of sense consciousness at the surface of the mind and experiencing total stillness within your greater Kelee is the goal of Step Two. Stillness is defined as a non-distracted, one-pointed awareness of self. It is achieved when there is an absence of thinking. If you are visualizing, trying to resolve an issue, planning activities, or distracted by the five physical senses while meditating, you are thinking and not doing Kelee meditation. After experiencing stillness, you return to full consciousness at the surface of the mind. Step Two should end after about three minutes.

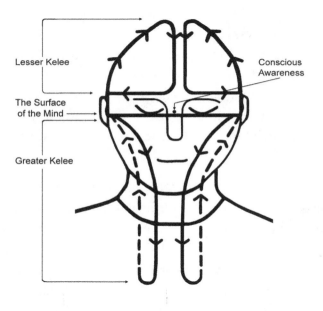

Lesser Kelee

Conscious Awareness

The Surface of the Mind

Greater Kelee

Overview of Kelee Meditation

Step Three

Upon returning from meditation (stillness), reflect on the quality of your practice through introspection and contemplation.

Introspection is when you look within your Kelee from the surface of the mind and reflect on the quality of your meditation. The introspection portion of Kelee meditation requires you to truthfully evaluate your meditation and is for retrospective and observational purposes.

Contemplation is when you ponder your observations. Pondering is viewing without an expectation of learning in this moment. Pondering is a form of mind function. This provides an opportunity for self-understanding. The time devoted to contemplation will teach you a great deal about yourself. *Questions to ask during contemplation:*

1. Can I mentally locate and feel my conscious awareness at the top of my head?
2. Could I mentally feel my conscious awareness as a plane of awareness relaxing down to the surface of my mind?
3. Did I have any thoughts in my lesser Kelee?
4. Could I feel my conscious awareness drop into the greater Kelee, and how detached did I feel from the surface of the mind?
5. Did I sense any compartments or images in the greater Kelee?
6. How one-pointed and still was I in the greater Kelee?
7. In an overall sense does my mind, nervous system, and body feel calmer?

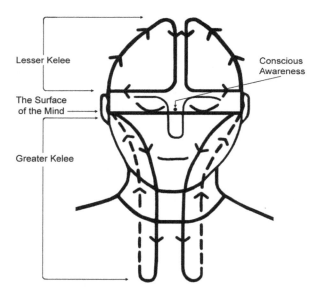

Overview of Kelee Meditation

Step Three (continued)

It is difficult to completely still your mind on command. The discipline of reaching stillness is an ongoing process. Excellence takes time. It is important that you are honest and kind when grading the quality of your meditation. The quality of stillness will improve with time and practice. As long as you sincerely put in the effort to help yourself, the results will come. Step Three of the Practice should be a minimum of five minutes.

The Time-Patience Equation

Quite often people ask, "Why is the time spent doing Kelee meditation so short?" The lesser Kelee is filled with tension from compartments and there is a time-density equation with the rate at which they will dissolve.

The rate that a compartment will break down will depend on the density of the compartment and the quality of your stillness. Two minutes of slowly moving through the lesser Kelee to the surface of the mind may seem like a short amount of time for a meditation technique to have any effect. However, meditating longer does not necessarily speed up the dissolution of compartments.

When you drop your conscious awareness into your greater Kelee, you may notice that the greater Kelee is non-linear and that there is no concept of time. It is intellectual brain function that makes time real and exist. In the non-linear experience of the greater Kelee, it's about the quality of being still. Do not pay attention to the amount of

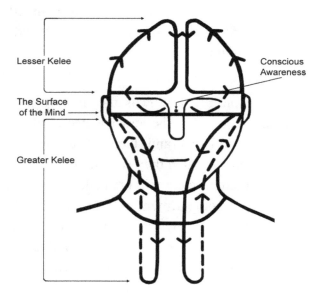

Lesser Kelee

Conscious Awareness

The Surface of the Mind

Greater Kelee

Overview of Kelee Meditation

The Time-Patience Equation (continued)

time you spend while in the greater Kelee. Your mental command of your biological clock will bring you back at about three minutes. The biological clock is an inherent awareness of time we all have within. After you have been practicing for a while, setting your biological clock will become an automatic response.

After being still for three minutes in the greater Kelee, you return to full awareness at the surface of the mind and start introspection and contemplation. This is the time to ponder what you have seen in your Kelee.

Note: Doing Kelee meditation will take patience. If you are not patient, then you are impatient and that leads to frustration and the creation of mental blocks (i.e., compartments).

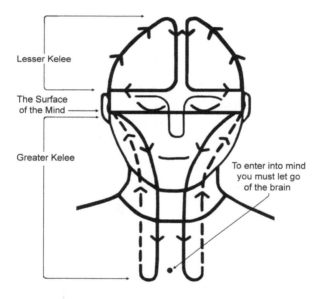

Lesser Kelee

The Surface of the Mind

Greater Kelee

To enter into mind you must let go of the brain

Chapter Fourteen

Effects of Kelee Meditation

The effects of Kelee meditation
are centered
in the thought that,
when the mind
is brought into harmony,
it will heal
the physical body.

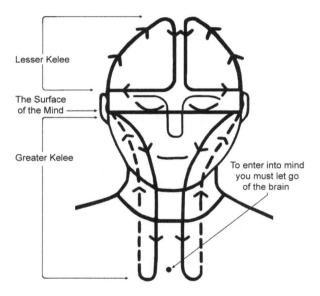

Lesser Kelee

The Surface
of the Mind

Greater Kelee

To enter into mind
you must let go
of the brain

Effects of Kelee Meditation

The three most detrimental influences on the physical body are stress, anxiety, and depression. To troubleshoot the body's major internal systems you must understand how these three mental disruptions affect the physical body.

Stress: Stress occurs when you feel unprepared to deal with life situations. It manifests as sensory overload on one's nervous system, which either leads into anxiety or depression, depending on how you deal with it. Stress can affect every system in the body. It can be dissipated by detaching into a calm mind that does not loop.

Anxiety: Anxiety manifests as excessive nervous energy in the central nervous system. It is when you have the energy to do something but lack the understanding of knowing what to do (i.e., you worry or become fearful). Anxiety can affect the nervous system and the entire physical body. Anxiety can be dissolved through Kelee meditation.

Depression: Depression manifests when you do not feel good about yourself and you turn on yourself. This causes a drop in electrochemical energy in the physical body and limits your mental ability because of a lack of energy. Depression can affect every system in the physical body. Depression can be dissolved through Kelee meditation.

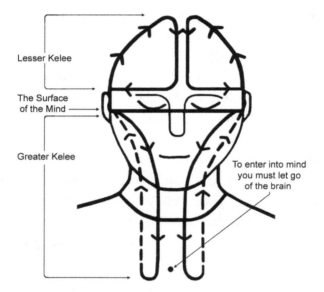

Lesser Kelee

The Surface of the Mind

Greater Kelee

To enter into mind you must let go of the brain

Effects of Kelee Meditation

Everything in being healthy in body and mind is about paying attention to all the contributing factors that promote good health. *Here are a few important areas to ponder:*

1. Do you get proper sleep?

2. Do you eat good food that promotes health?

3. Do you get enough physical exercise?

4. Do you mentally care about yourself?

5. Do you ever try to escape your problems instead of facing them?

6. Do you ever treat others wrongly with negative thoughts?

7. Do you ever ask yourself who you are, why you are here, and where you are going?

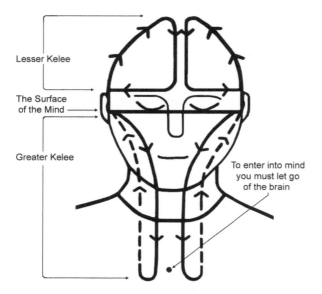

Lesser Kelee

The Surface
of the Mind

Greater Kelee

To enter into mind
you must let go
of the brain

Effects of Kelee Meditation

The following pages outline the basic understanding of how your thoughts and feelings affect each of the human body's systems listed below (i.e., the mind-body connection) and how these systems relate to stress, anxiety, and depression.

1. Immune system

2. Nervous system

3. Cardiovascular system

4. Respiratory system

5. Digestive system

6. Endocrine system

7. Skeletal system

8. Other effects

   a. Nutrition

   b. Sleep

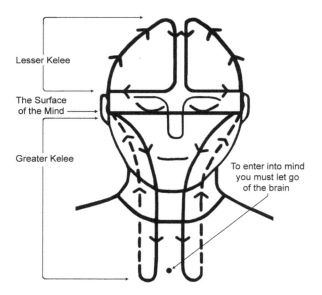

Lesser Kelee

The Surface
of the Mind

Greater Kelee

To enter into mind
you must let go
of the brain

Effects of Kelee Meditation
on the Immune System

Your immune system is your first line of defense in the human body. In early primitive man it was about "survival of the fittest." Those who were the most intelligent and the most physically fit (as determined by the strongest genes i.e., deoxyribonucleic acid [DNA]) survived.

Today it is still your DNA in the physical that's important. However, it is not the most intelligent today that will dominate but the wisest, more aware beings that will lead the way. This wisdom is harmony of being and is found through understanding not only how to develop intelligence in the intellect, but also through perception into deeper states of mind.

The biggest culprit in crashing your immune system is an unstable conscious awareness. In an outward sense, without understanding the consequences of your actions, lack of awareness occurs, which causes stress and mental disharmony. In an inward sense, without awareness of mind, you can be overtaken by your compartments, which can crash your immune system. Stress, anxiety, and depression are usually involved here.

Compartments can drain the energy from your immune system twenty-four hours a day, seven days a week. All of this can be reversed with Kelee meditation.

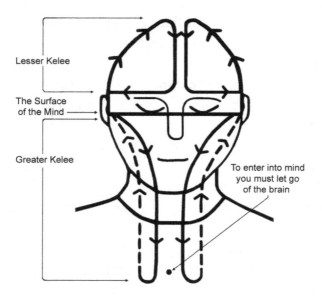

Lesser Kelee

The Surface
of the Mind

Greater Kelee

To enter into mind
you must let go
of the brain

Effects of Kelee Meditation
on the Nervous System

The nervous system is vital in providing a connection to how you feel. There are two ways in which you can feel via the nervous system—physically and mentally.

The physical way of feeling occurs via your pain and pleasure response and is a secondary point of awareness. However, when it comes to your mental feeling sense, then a much deeper and more complex experience happens. This is because of emotions realized in your primary point—your mind.

The nervous system is subject to stress because of excess stimulation. When this happens you hear phrases like, "I am fried" or "My nerves are shot," and so on!

Despite the advances of technology, seeing a tree on a computer screen does not feel the same as a real tree. Computer games have a different affect on your nervous system than playing games outdoors. Moderation is the key to managing stress with technology.

The nervous system is also subject to anxiety and depression. When the nervous system is anxious it is shaky, and when depressed it is achy. Stress, anxiety, and depression can be changed by dissolving compartments. It is through detachment of mind and by entering into more harmonious states of mind that you can calm and balance the nervous system.

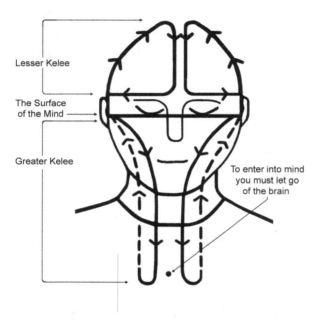

Lesser Kelee

The Surface
of the Mind

Greater Kelee

To enter into mind
you must let go
of the brain

Effects of Kelee Meditation
on the Cardiovascular System

Your cardiovascular system has both a physical and a mental component. When you talk about your heart, you do not segregate it to just the physical heart. There is also your heart associated with emotions. The brain is more associated with your physical heart, whereas your mind has more to do with emotions that can affect your heart.

Have you ever heard the phrases, "My heart just sank" or "My heart is heavy"? When this happens, emotions can affect your physical heart. Have you ever had a compartmentalized fear that is not a fight-or-flight type of fear (i.e., being chased by a bear) make your heart race? Learning to not fear non fight-or-flight fears (i.e., compartments) is an effect of Kelee meditation.

There is an intimate connection between how the emotions of the mind can affect the physical heart. It is a known fact that stress can affect the heart in physical ways. With Kelee meditation, the mind can calm stress on command. When you pay attention, you will notice that when your heart is warm with beautiful emotion, your physical heart feels healthier.

A happy heart is what supports the physical heart and can do wonders for your entire being, and that feeling is felt in the greater Kelee.

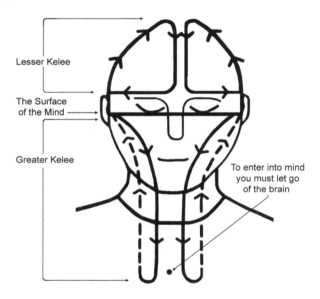

Lesser Kelee

The Surface
of the Mind

Greater Kelee

To enter into mind
you must let go
of the brain

Effects of Kelee Meditation
on the Respiratory System

Our respiratory system, for the most part, is controlled by the autonomic nervous system. However, there are times when compartmentalized emotion can alter one's breathing. For instance, a strong compartmentalized emotion can make someone hold their breath or breathe faster (hyperventilate) for no apparent reason. When you are stressed, you tend to not breathe. When you have anxiety, you tend to breathe faster and more often, yet still feel short of breath. When you are depressed, you don't care to breathe at all.

The respiratory system can also be compromised by the sheer tension in our nervous system, which is held in place by deep unconscious emotion. As you delve deep into the Kelee, your conscious awareness will uncover many stationary compartments that have been operating and compromising your health for a long time.

The term, breath of life, is very real. It is a known fact that most people do not breathe enough. There are also many lifestyle reasons for not breathing properly, such as a lack of self-awareness and sedentary jobs. There can be many reasons for this—study your own.

The autonomic nervous system may unconsciously function to assist you in maneuvering through life, but there is more you can do to be healthy. It is through the awareness of mind that the mind-body connection is realized and understood.

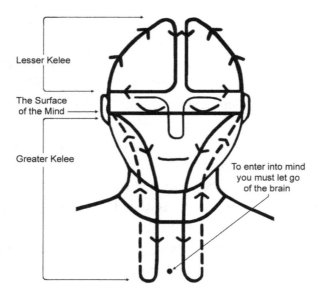

Lesser Kelee

The Surface
of the Mind

Greater Kelee

To enter into mind
you must let go
of the brain

Effects of Kelee Meditation
on the Digestive System

Your digestive system has an intimate connection with the mind. First and foremost, everything you put in your mouth is because of you. All eating disorders have to do with the mind and can also be solved by it. Those who are more aware and educated eat a better quality food, whereas those who are unaware and uneducated eat without a regard for nutrition.

We must ask ourselves, "What determines what you put in your mouth? And is it your conscious awareness, or just a physical craving?" Understanding the mind is not only about what you put in your mouth, but how you feel emotionally—good and bad—when you eat.

The world is filled with stress and when this stress affects our digestive system, problems occur. When our mind cannot detach from stress, it becomes our body's. When the stomach is stressed, it tends to release too much stomach acid thereby causing a problem. When the small intestines become hard and rigid, the nutrients in food are not properly absorbed. As food moves into the large intestines another stress related problem can occur—constipation. When one cannot mentally relax, the large intestines cannot function naturally. When one cannot eliminate waste by regular bowel movements, toxins in the physical body accumulate.

When one eats good quality food and feels good about it, proper physiological and mental nutrition is achieved. Remember, when the mind is relaxed, the physical body follows suit.

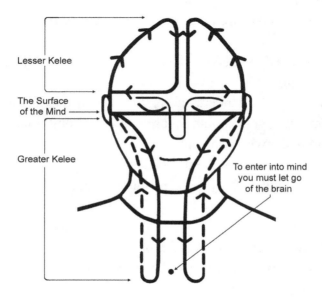

Lesser Kelee

The Surface
of the Mind

Greater Kelee

To enter into mind
you must let go
of the brain

Effects of Kelee Meditation
on the Endocrine System

Our endocrine system is an intense system in the human body. Its job is to facilitate communication between cells and to regulate body functions via the release of hormones. Components of the endocrine system include hormone-producing glands, such as the hypothalamus, pituitary, thyroid, adrenal glands, and reproductive organs. Each of these glands and organs in the endocrine system produce different types of hormones that perform different functions.

Why the endocrine system can be problematic is because negative feelings can interfere with the regulation of hormones. How many people do you know that have had hormones run their thoughts and their life?

Let's look at the hormones associated with sexuality. When you have too much sex, or not enough sex, problems can occur. Then bring in passion and one's search for the experience of love, and things can become much more complex. If the endocrine system is not balanced with harmony of mind, many problems can occur.

How do you regulate all of these hormones? It happens by achieving balance in the electrochemical process via harmony of mind. This harmony of mind begins with calming the mind. It is a calm mind that balances the electrochemical process of the physical body and the emotions associated with the endocrine system.

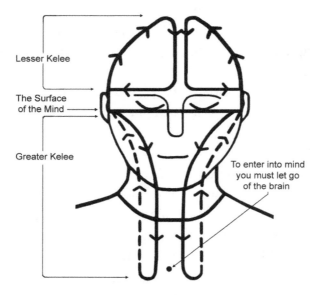

Lesser Kelee

The Surface
of the Mind

Greater Kelee

To enter into mind
you must let go
of the brain

Effects of Kelee Meditation
on the Skeletal System

You need a skeletal system for many reasons. One reason is for survival. Survival of the fittest is not just about having brute strength and good DNA. It is the most aware, perceptive beings that will ultimately lead the way on our evolutionary process from *homo sapiens* to *homo novus,* which means freedom from instrumentality.

The skeletal system is what keeps your body in a structure that is functional; it protects your vital organs, such as the heart, brain, and lungs. It also enables you to move and do all of the things that humans like to do. The skeletal system is mainly associated with the physical aspect of life, but there is a much deeper aspect associated with the mind.

At the deepest level, the essence of the mind permeates every bone in your body. Without the sentience of mind, the physical body has no life. Because the skeletal system produces red and white blood cells in our bone marrow, it is extremely important that your essence at the deepest level is healthy. That occurs by way of developing harmony of mind.

When stress, anxiety, and depression are prevalent, it puts a drain on this system. This is a drain you can learn to eliminate through Kelee meditation.

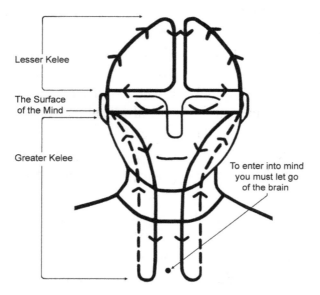

Lesser Kelee

The Surface
of the Mind

Greater Kelee

To enter into mind
you must let go
of the brain

Effects of Kelee Meditation
on Nutrition

Nutrition from food is basically a physical form of your energy system. It is very important to understand the relationship between our electrochemical energy and mind. When the base energy of the physical body is weak, it affects the higher functions of the mind. If you are to learn, your energy must be stable.

This stability can occur on two levels. There is the motivational energy (from food) associated with the intellect, and on a deeper level, there is the inspirational energy (from mind). Whenever you do not feel well (either on a physical or mental level), you suffer.

All you need to know about good nutrition is written and available, and can be found with research on your part. The question is why would you have resistance to listening to what will help you to feel better. These are the mental blocks (i.e., compartments) that occur in the Kelee.

The physical body and brain are like your car, and the mind is the driver. Look at food as your fuel. It is wise to use the highest grade of fuel. At the same time, it is also wise to be a driver alert with awareness of mind to limit distractions, which cause most accidents.

The finest minds in the world are the ones that pay attention. A pure genius is characterized by having a focused undistracted mind. This is when you are in primary point of mind and your attention is then fully focused on a second point.

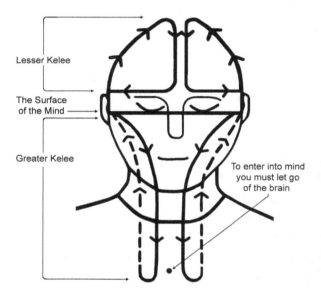

Lesser Kelee

The Surface
of the Mind

Greater Kelee

To enter into mind
you must let go
of the brain

Effects of Kelee Meditation
on Sleep

Sleep is your primary form of regeneration and extremely important in maintaining health. The biggest problem people have with sleep is not being able to sleep. This is because one cannot stop the thinking process of the brain even when one wants to. The brain can run independent of the mind; however, it does so without regard for your health and well-being. The question becomes, why can't you shut down this thinking process when you want to? It's because the brain and compartments have more control than you do. So who is in control of your life?

The primary form of regeneration should come from stillness of the mind in the greater Kelee and learning to detach from the thinking process. When you have excessive thinking, it's because you have no resolution from your troubling thoughts. You cannot let go of a thought until you understand it. This is basic human nature. Everyone will have to come to terms with this understanding one day.

If you decide to mentally block out or ignore a non-understood thought, it electrochemically deposits (i.e., compartmentalizes) in the Kelee and "baggage" is formed. As you have more of these unresolved thoughts in your Kelee, the result is fragmentation, which leads to frustration and sleeplessness. This is all reversed when you can enter into peace of mind found in the greater Kelee.

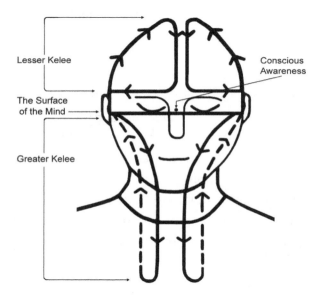

Chapter Fifteen

Ins and Outs of Kelee Meditation

*The ins and outs
will explain what happens
as a result of doing Kelee meditation.
Doing Kelee meditation
opens you
to a firsthand learning experience
of how your mind works
in practicality not theory.*

Ins and Outs
of Kelee Meditation

1. A healthy physical body is supported by a healthy clear mind via Kelee meditation. The depth of the relationship between the mind and the body is integral and cannot be separated, except by death. The mind associated with sentience and the physical body associated with viability coexist together. Every person alive will have to accept the fact that our thoughts affect our actions and our actions affect our lives.

The depth of how our thoughts help us or hinder us is a study of our mind's relationship with the Kelee. The finite aspect of the brain and intellect and the infinite experience of the mind will take you to places that you have never seen before. This is the human quest and the purpose of life—to realize the unknown through complete self-understanding of everything.

2. The side effects of Kelee meditation are actually benefits; a still mind balances the electrochemical energy of the physical body naturally. The major side effect of Kelee meditation is processing. Processing starts when you detach from brain function and enter into mind function.

There are three ways to deal with any type of dysfunction. One way to deal with dysfunction is through developing and using coping mechanisms, which can take a lot of unconscious mental energy to maintain. Another way is to loop with dysfunction, which is often very uncomfortable. The final way is to detach from dysfunction and begin

Ins and Outs
of Kelee Meditation

2. processing, which is only temporary. This is the worst side effect of Kelee meditation. However, once an electrochemical compartment is dissolved, its physiological and mental effect on you is gone forever.

3. One of the first observations that you will notice as a result of Kelee meditation is that things that used to bother you, no longer do. The first time this happens, you will be startled. You'll ask yourself, "Shouldn't that have affected me?" But it does not.

4. Another observation from Kelee meditation that you will notice is that all of nature will become more vibrant, such as the clouds in the sky, the many shades of green in the trees, birds and butterflies flying by, and feeling the wind on your face like you've never experienced before. This happens as a result of your mind seeing through your brain.

5. The rewards received from Kelee meditation are experienced as a happy, unworried mind. This unworried mind happens as a result of detachment from troubling thoughts. When the conscious awareness is open to the Kelee, freedom and genuine happiness occur.

6. Kelee meditation slows the degeneration process typically associated with aging. Each time you still your mind, your mental and physical body rejuvenates. When the nervous system and the heart rate are calmed and slowed

Ins and Outs
of Kelee Meditation

6. *(cont.)* down, regeneration occurs, but without requiring sleep. The deepest form of regeneration is from a still mind. A mind that is sleeping can also be restless, and therefore, can limit regeneration. It is from a still mind that sleep patterns can deepen over time. This occurs by eliminating compartments that refuse to sleep and disturb restfulness at night.

7. Efficiency at work will increase because your conscious awareness is not scattered with too many thoughts from compartments. This naturally improves your ability to focus without distraction. When you are more efficient, you gain self-confidence and enjoy your work. You also have more time with your own thoughts because you are not always stressed from inefficiency.

Your work stops being separate from your life because you enjoy what you do. Work is no longer disliked. Happiness is worth more than money, and yet, you can actually enjoy your job and value being paid for your efforts.

8. A deeper self-awareness enhances relationships at home and work. You develop and gain the ability to give from your heart without expecting anything in return. When you feel good within, everything in your life gets better. A deeper connection to life is the result from your newly developing awareness, opening you to experiences that allow you to feel all that life has to offer.

Ins and Outs
of Kelee Meditation

9. It is not unusual to feel a small drop in physical energy after beginning Kelee meditation. Your calming mind begins to wean off adrenaline-based, anxious energy. After a short period of time, your energy level will stabilize into an overall feeling of calmness. You will have a new self-understanding of stable electrochemical energy.

As your mind opens and deepens to new levels of energy efficiency, you do not burn energy wastefully. You move with grace instead of haste. You develop finesse.

10. When you begin to drop the walls of resistance in your mind, you may feel some emotional discomfort as you process out compartments. Once a compartment is gone, you will not experience that particular dysfunction again. This is hard to believe but can be experienced. When you think you should be triggered and nothing happens, you will witness something amazing—the absence of dysfunction from compartmentalization.

11. When you are processing, be good to yourself. You may want to sleep more than usual. This is normal. Give yourself a mental health day, if you can. If not, pace yourself throughout your day. Processing is not exactly fun. However, the alternative is worse and continually repeats throughout your life. The right thought to have while processing is how good you will feel when your dysfunctional compartment is gone.

Ins and Outs
of Kelee Meditation

12. From time to time you will experience physiological effects when processing, such as headaches, nausea, low energy, depression, or anxiety. If a compartment was linked with physical discomfort at the time it was formed, it will mimic the same response when it is being processed out. Any physical discomfort will cease when the electrochemical compartment is dissolved. The mind's effect on the physical body is called psychosomatism. When the mind causes a psychosomatic disorder, the mind can reverse it.

13. Stress from fragmented energy, anxiety from too much energy, and depression from not having enough energy will eventually disappear as you continue practicing Kelee meditation. These three big deterrents to humanity can be changed with some work on your part. Ironically, the work that is required is to learn to do nothing with your mind—still your mind.

As you do Kelee meditation, those around you will notice the changes in how you look and feel. This is one of the hallmarks of Kelee meditation. You will feel lighter as compartments dissipate and the results become noticeably visible to others, as a vibrant healthier you emerges.

14. As negative, energy-draining compartments are deleted, the immune system is boosted and freed to function at optimal efficiency. The amount of energy that compartments drain is enormous. They operate twenty-four hours a day,

Ins and Outs
of Kelee Meditation

14. seven days a week, and even when we sleep. Ponder the reverse of this process and you will be inspired when you are not being drained. It is a known fact that when you are in a bad mood due to compartments, you get very little done that is of quality. When the brain and the mind work in harmony, whatever you are doing or wherever you are, is amazing.

15. Elation occurs when the space occupied by dysfunction is replaced by the true nature of your being. Elation is a reward for your diligence and manifests as a potent, natural, euphoric feeling which stimulates the release of endorphins and the body's natural tranquilizers. This beautiful feeling of elation is felt from the essence of your being and is often referred to as "big sky mind" because of its open blue appearance. This unobstructed space in your Kelee is the place where true happiness originates.

16. If you are slow to wake up in the morning or too tired at bedtime, do Kelee meditation whenever possible; however, the goal is to become accustomed to a morning and evening routine. When doing Kelee meditation sit with your spine erect. Do not do Kelee meditation lying down—it's too easy to go to sleep. Stillness of mind is not sleep! Sleep is when you let go of consciousness. Stillness is when you are conscious at a still point with an awareness of nothing. This is the primary point of mind without a second point to think about. You are conscious and aware of nothing.

Ins and Outs
of Kelee Meditation

17. If you are falling asleep while meditating, you are either too tired or too relaxed. When your conscious awareness is too relaxed, it will spread out and wander. Refocus by pulling all of your awareness to a pinpoint within you. The sleep/stillness line of distinction takes time to master. Do Kelee meditation to the best of your ability and consider it a success because you did it.

18. Set your biological clock for about three minutes before you drop into your greater Kelee. This becomes automatic after the first few times. This is the same clock in your mind that can wake you at the same time every morning. Setting your biological clock happens by repetition or by thought command. While you are in the non-linear space of the greater Kelee, there is no existence of time. That is why the biological clock is needed.

19. The time you are in your Kelee is not the time to investigate what you see and experience! If you are thinking or drifting off, your conscious awareness cannot be still. The absence of thought-form images allows stillness to occur and is the objective of Kelee meditation. If you are observing while in your practice, you will not be still and will not proceed into deeper states of awareness. It is by being still in your greater Kelee that the mind continues to open over time. The time to investigate your Kelee and your thoughts is when you come back from your practice. This is done at the surface of the mind.

Ins and Outs
of Kelee Meditation

20. Keep a journal to record your experience after your practice. This will be a record of your personal growth and development. What happens in your practice is what is happening in your mind. Remember this! There will always be a record of thought activity when you finish your practice. After your practice is the time to write down your thoughts and ponder why you have them.

Your development is to understand your thoughts. If you never study your thoughts, how will you learn from them? Keep in mind, in order to study thoughts that you don't understand, you must be in mind function. This is the only way for you to realize why they are there. Over time, you will be amazed at how much you will learn about your thought process. Writing down your thoughts is a way to bring the intellectual process in harmony with the mind.

21. Do Kelee meditation even when you do not feel like it; this is when you need to do it the most. If you miss your practice in the morning for some reason, find a quiet safe place to do your practice when you have a break. Doing your practice is like going to work to get paid. If you do not do your practice, you do not get paid in clarity and peace of mind. When your practice is no longer work, you will enjoy doing it. Is it not better to be relaxed and still than to be stressed and hurried?

22. Once you understand the basic principles of the Kelee, you will have a way to understand the mysteries of thought

Ins and Outs
of Kelee Meditation

22. *(cont.)* and emotion, including their effects on your mind and body. The evolution and depth of experience that you will discover in Kelee meditation is infinite; ironically it just takes time and patience to understand the infinite nature of your being.

23. There are three disciplines of Kelee meditation:

Meditation: This is the time to learn how to develop stillness of mind at one point in the greater Kelee. The goal is to have an awareness of nothing, which is defined as having one point of awareness without the distraction from a second point of observation.

Introspection: As you come out of your practice, your still point opens to a second point of observation. This is when perfect receptivity is achieved. This is the time to look back in your memory to recall what you remember from your practice. Your mind will have a record of everything that is not still.

Contemplation: This is the time used to study why you have the thoughts that you do. This focus of attention can direct you to areas of interest for you to study. You can then analyze them from brain or observe them from mind freely, without predetermination.

24. There are three P's of Kelee meditation:

Practice: Without entering into mind, stillness will not occur. Stillness opens up to clarity and detachment.

Ins and Outs
of Kelee Meditation

24. Without detachment, compartments will not dissolve, thereby blocking your development and learning process.

Persistence: Without persistence, you will not have continuity—the process whereby you mentally grow and evolve into deeper and more harmonious states of mind.

Patience: Without patience, you are impatient. This hinders the learning process because you cannot sit still to be still. The way to master patience is to be in mind. The mind is non-linear and does not know what time is, therefore you are patient.

25. Do Kelee meditation for ten minutes in the morning and ten minutes in the evening. The purpose of the first five minutes is to be as still of thought as you can. The purpose of the next five minutes is to study your thoughts upon returning to full awareness. Stillness opens you up to clarity, and clarity opens you up to the understanding and realization of life experiences.

26. If you have not given Kelee meditation a solid effort for at least six months, you have not given yourself a chance to know what a clear mind feels like. After all, what kind of a degree, that has any depth of understanding, can you honestly obtain with just six months of study?

The understanding of all your life experiences will take time to study. The study will start with your conscious

Ins and Outs
of Kelee Meditation

26. *(cont.)* thoughts and issues, leading into your subconscious, and with extended study, into the deeper realms of your unconscious. Your life is affected by many influences, it would be wise to know what affects you and why, if you are to attain the fulfillment of your goals in this life. This exploration of mind will be the deepest, most fascinating experience of your life. Are you not curious to explore what moves you?

Keep in mind that Kelee meditation does not require a lot of time. Ten minutes out of twenty-four hours is less than one percent of your day to devote to clarity and the direction of your entire life.

*The Kelee meditation practice
calls for dedication
of studying your mind,
with living in mind as the goal
and happiness as your reward.*

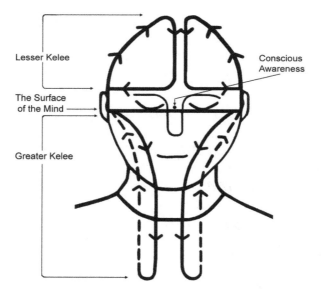

Chapter Sixteen

How to Do Kelee Meditation

The hardest thing
about Kelee meditation
is doing it twice a day.
If you do not do Kelee meditation,
nothing will happen.
You must do the work
to get results.
You must practice
to get out of brain function
and into mind function.
Practice does make perfect.

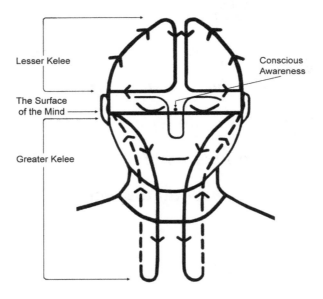

Lesser Kelee

The Surface
of the Mind

Greater Kelee

Conscious
Awareness

How to Do
Kelee Meditation

Step One: *Approximately two minutes.*

Sit down, get comfortable, and begin relaxing brain activity. Mentally feel your conscious awareness at the top of your head and mentally relax this horizontal plane of awareness through both hemispheres of your brain, ultimately settling at the surface of the mind. At the surface of the mind, be consciously relaxed, but not thinking.

Step Two: *Approximately three minutes.*

After relaxing at the surface of the mind, mentally allow your conscious awareness to drop below the surface of the mind, to a still point within the greater Kelee. The goal is to let go of sense consciousness and experience total stillness for about three minutes.

Note: Before dropping from the surface of the mind into the greater Kelee, set your biological clock to come back to complete awareness in about three minutes.

Step Three: *Approximately five minutes.*

After experiencing stillness, return to full consciousness at the surface of the mind and reflect on what you noticed about your practice. Do not bolt into the day. The goal is to do Kelee meditation for ten minutes in the morning and evening to the best of your ability and get into the experience of life.

Recommendation: Keep a journal to record experiences and progress. You may think you will remember everything, but many subtle gems of wisdom and growth will be forgotten if not written down.

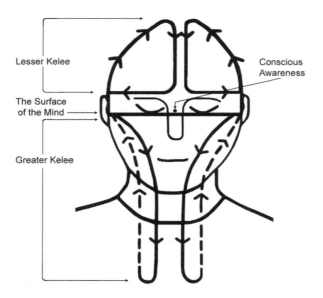

Lesser Kelee

Conscious
Awareness

The Surface
of the Mind

Greater Kelee

Conceptual Medical Model of Kelee Meditation

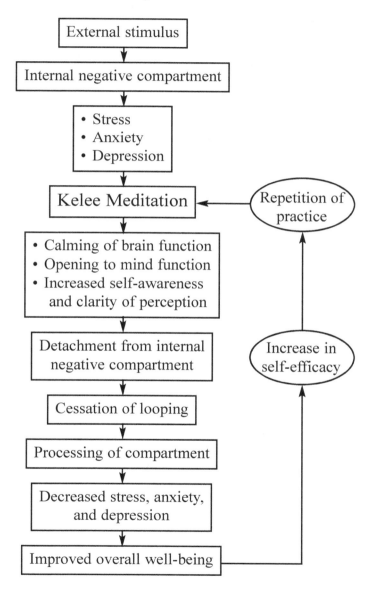

External stimulus

Internal negative compartment

- Stress
- Anxiety
- Depression

Kelee Meditation ← Repetition of practice

- Calming of brain function
- Opening to mind function
- Increased self-awareness and clarity of perception

Detachment from internal negative compartment

Cessation of looping

Processing of compartment

Decreased stress, anxiety, and depression

Improved overall well-being

Increase in self-efficacy

Never underestimate the power of calmness to start the process of health and regeneration. Stress does not allow the nervous system to work properly. It is calmness of mind that soothes the physical body into healing.

To heal, we must calm ourselves and allow ourselves to be peaceful.

"Be at peace
with yourself.
If you are not at peace
with yourself,
you are at peace
with nothing."

—*Ron W. Rathbun*

About the Author

Ron W. Rathbun's fascination with human emotions and the mind stems back to his teenage years. Ron was enrolled at a community college to begin studying psychology when he met Dr. Eugene C. Larr, a retired professor from Cal Tech in Pasadena, California, who had two PhDs and three master's degrees. After meeting this man, Ron knew he had found his teacher—the one who would become his mentor. Ron studied and consulted privately with his mentor about the inner workings of the Kelee for twenty-eight years, until Dr. Larr's passing in 2006.

Ron's career as a teacher began in 1985 and in January of 1993, he began teaching Kelee meditation. He has taught Kelee meditation to people from all walks of life, many of whom are physicians. In September of 2008, The University of California, San Diego Institutional Review Board granted full approval to begin a medical study to measure the change and effects of Kelee meditation on patients suffering from stress, anxiety, and depression.

Ron Rathbun continues to research and study the effects of the mind on the immune system and nervous system in relation to healing the physiology of the body. Ron teaches that within you is the ability to bring about anything your mind can dream of, all that's needed is inspiration, clarity, and time. All of these gifts are within you all. Allow your conscious awareness to open to your Kelee and it will begin to happen.

Contact Us

What each person brings to the world is what they have within. It is our mission to offer, to all those who are seeking, a way to internally heal one's own mind through Kelee meditation. For it is the condition of one's Kelee that influences one's emotional and physical health and wellness.

The Kelee Foundation is a 501(c)(3) nonprofit, tax-exempt organization. It is generously funded by the donations of all those who recognize the health benefits of a clear mind. Please feel free to contact us if you are interested in learning more.

Web site: www.thekelee.org

Facebook: The Kelee Foundation

CPSIA information can be obtained
at www.ICGtesting.com
Printed in the USA
LVHW111030040621
689359LV00004B/184